AFFORDABLE HEALTHY FOOD

THE ESSENTIAL NUTRITION GUIDE FOR
ACHIEVING OPTIMAL HEALTH ON A BUDGET

RENEE AFRYKA, M.S.
REGISTERED DIETITIAN NUTRITIONIST

Affordable Healthy Food:
The Essential Nutrition Guide for Achieving Optimal Health on a Budget

Copyright © 2025 by Renee Afryka

This book is not intended as a substitute for the medical advice of physicians. The reader should regularly consult a physician in matters relating to their health, particularly with respect to any symptoms that may require diagnosis or medical attention.

All rights reserved. This book or any portion thereof may not be reproduced or used in any manner whatsoever without the express written permission of the publisher except for the use of brief quotations in a book review.

ISBN 979-8-303-55375-0

To God, you already know,

and

To my powerful soulmate, husband, and best friend,
who challenges me and opens my world every single day.
Thank you, Imani.

TABLE OF CONTENTS

Introduction. 1

PART 1:
THE TOOLS – Food Preparation Methods, Meals, and More 13
    Chapter 1: Easy Food Preparation Methods 13
    Chapter 2: Food Savings Pro Tips. 37
    Chapter 3: Staple Foods to Have on Hand. 57
    Chapter 4: Drinks 61
    Chapter 5: Snacks 75
    Chapter 6: Breakfast 99
    Chapter 7: Lunch. 109
    Chapter 8: Dinner 119
    Chapter 9: Eating Out on a Budget. 137
    Chapter 10: Sample Grocery List and Menu 143

PART 2:
THE KNOWLEDGE – Nutrition Basics 147
    Chapter 11: Why Do You Want to Be Healthy? 149
    Chapter 12: Calories 155
    Chapter 13: Decoding the Mysteries of The Nutrition Facts
                  Label and Ingredients List 165
    Chapter 14: Carbohydrates 183
    Chapter 15: Fats. 207
    Chapter 16: Proteins 231
    Chapter 17: Vitamins, Minerals and Phytonutrients.. 239
    Chapter 18: Nutrition Questions Answered 251

PART 3:
THE WORK – Taking Care of You 263
    Chapter 19: Relax and Give Yourself a Break 265
    Chapter 20: More Stress Management Techniques 291

PART 4:
THE SUPPORT – Resources Available for You 299
    Chapter 21: Food Assistance and Other Resources 301
    Chapter 22: Putting It All Together 313

    Endnotes.. 315
    Index... 321

INTRODUCTION

If healthy eating and wellness are your goals but feel like a burden you don't have the money for, the time to think about, or the energy to figure out, this book is for you. I have helped thousands of people with limited incomes achieve their health goals, and I want to help you too.

I don't blame you for feeling that healthy eating is financially out of your reach. Our cultural narrative is that healthy eating is too expensive. I say that it does not have to be. In fact, I will show you evidence that healthy eating can be much more affordable than unhealthy eating and equally delicious.

You may also feel like healthy eating is out of reach because of all the confusing nutrition news in the media. One day, we are told that a certain food is good for us, and the next day, it is not. The key to navigating this conflicting news is understanding the basics—nutrition, and cooking—that you will learn here in parts one and two.

Being healthy does not mean extreme diets and strict rules. It can also be about small steps. There was a time when we looked down on a person who ordered a double cheeseburger, a large fry, and a diet drink. We would say things like, "What's the point?" With that mentality, taking small steps was stigmatized. But what if I told you that ordering something like water or unsweetened iced tea, even with the double cheeseburger and large fry, makes a big difference and costs the same or less?[1] We will destigmatize the "small" steps approach and appreciate them for what they are: healthy choices that make a big difference.

Don't give up on your hopes of eating a nutritious diet and feeling your best. Have hope that you can eat well even if you don't have an endless budget, much time, or cooking skills. Incorporating more nutritious foods may take a little shifting around of your daily routine. It also may mean that you expand your horizons a little. Being willing to try new foods and different versions of the foods we don't like can open up an entire world.

Brussels sprouts were vegetables that I hated, but I realized that I just didn't like the boiled versions. When I started roasting them with about a tablespoon of oil and salt, they tasted much better. In fact, they are one of my favorite vegetables now. They are also one of the most nutrient-rich vegetables and only cost about $0.50 per serving.

I teach easy, affordable cooking classes, and I cannot tell you the number of times I have heard someone say something like, "I normally don't like XYZ vegetable/food, but this is good. I would make this myself!" Don't get me wrong; there will always be foods that we don't like, no matter how they are prepared. If that is the case, leave those foods be, but just be open to new and different.

Also, you don't have to give up your favorite food if you don't want to. Instead, you can gradually add new foods to what you and your family currently eat. Take things step-by-step. Scientific evidence suggests that when you break down your goals into smaller, realistic steps, you are more likely to achieve those goals.[2] Embrace eating the celery sticks that come with the chicken wings. Yep, it counts, even if you eat

> Be open to trying new things or to trying old things in new ways, and the world of delicious, affordable, and nutritious eating will open up.

the chicken wings, we'll get to that later. It's another small step that makes a big difference.

We are also going to go a little deeper into this healthy-eating-on-a-budget thing than just discussing cooking and nutrition. I don't know about you, but when I'm sad, I go for ice cream. Oh, who am I kidding, I also go for ice cream when I am happy, watching a movie, and all of that. We choose the foods we eat sometimes because of our mood, stress, or just because we want them. But some not-so-obvious reasons we choose certain foods are because of the environment others create for us (think commercials, images, smells, product placements) and the internal mental environment we create for ourselves (think self-talk).

Many of us are unaware of the amount of negative self-talk—food and non-food-related—we feed ourselves daily. We say things like, "I shouldn't be eating this; that's why I am so fat," "I am too lazy," and "Why did I do/eat that?" "I will never achieve my life/health goal, so why try?" "I am fifty years old and haven't accomplished anything," and "Why should they pick me? What have I done?" Talking to ourselves this way can affect our life choices, including our food choices. In part three of this book, we will turn that negativity around by practicing positive self-talk and learning to be kind to ourselves. Stop for a second and think about what it means to be kind to yourself.

This book provides activities that encourage us to practice being kind to ourselves. I'm talking about the genuine "I love myself," "I don't care how many mistakes I've made," or "I believe that I deserve it" kind of kindness.

We will also deal with the stress that impacts our food choices. Sometimes, there is something we can do about the stress in our lives—it's just that we may forget to step back, take a moment, and problem-solve. We don't typically bring stress and self-talk to the party when we discuss healthy eating, but we will be here.

We will cover food/cooking, nutrition, taking care of you, and, finally, food assistance. If you need a little extra help, you may be eligible for financial/food assistance. Some programs don't have eligibility requirements at all. You just walk in, and the food is available for you. You will find out more about these resources in part four.

What Does It Mean to Be a "Healthy Food"?

Ask different people, "What is a healthy diet?" and you will get different answers. We should be on the same page, so for this book, a healthy diet allows an individual to achieve optimal health. That means putting food inside you designed to make the body's systems operate at full capacity. A healthy diet will give you the best brain, heart, skin, kidney, liver, and lung health. It provides optimal hormone balance and the best infection and disease-fighting system, combating cancers, dementia, and even viruses like Covid-19. It will also provide high energy levels, pain relief, good emotional/mental health, an overall physical sensation of feeling good, and more.

While there are some fundamentals to healthy eating, in general, my "healthy diet" is not always going to be your "healthy diet," and your "healthy diet" is not always going to be my "healthy diet." This is why paying attention to how your body reacts to specific foods, food combinations, eating times, and more is important. More on that later.

> A "healthy food," for the purposes of this book, is a food that promotes optimal health while doing no harm.

If a healthy diet is a diet that promotes optimal health, then "healthy food," for the purposes of this book, is food that supports optimal health while doing no harm.

I am one of those professionals who believes in classifying foods as healthy or unhealthy—good or bad even. In some instances where nothing else is available, that "unhealthy" food might provide carbohydrates, protein, or fats that are important for survival, but overall, they do not promote optimal health. In fact, eating those "unhealthy" foods every day can cause the type of harm that is responsible for some of the health problems and disparities that we have in this country and around the world.

Table 1 characterizes foods commonly eaten in the United States as healthy or unhealthy. These designations are chosen based on my expertise. This is not agreed upon by the scientific, medical, nutrition, and dietetics community; however, it might remove some of the confusion around these foods and help us make healthier food choices.

— TABLE 1 —
HEALTHY VS. UNHEALTHY FOODS

CATEGORY	RECOMMENDATION	FOODS		
1: Healthy	Consume liberally (several times a day)	Vegetables Fruits Beans Lentils Nuts	Seeds Quinoa Millet Oats Herbs Spices	Water Tea
2: Healthy with some concern; not necessary for optimal health	Consume regularly (limit to once a day for most people)	Organic milk Yogurt Cottage Cheese Brown rice 100% Whole Grains (unsweetened)	Tofu Chicken Turkey Fish Eggs	Cacao/cocoa Coffee Raw honey Molasses Real maple syrup
3: Unhealthy with redeeming qualities	Consume in moderation	White rice White pasta White bread Cereals Plant-based milks*	Cheese Meat substitutes Ketchup BBQ sauce	Agave syrup* Raw/Turbinado Sugar Stevia*
4: Unhealthy with no redeeming qualities	Save for a special rare indulgence	Baked goods Fried foods Red meat Pork Artificial sweeteners White sugar Mayo	Ultra-processed foods (potato chips, cheesy snack crackers, cookies, sweets, protein bars, etc.)	Processed meats (salami, bacon, sausage, pepperoni), Sugary drinks (soda, sports/energy drinks, flavored lemonades, etc.)

*I included these items in the "unhealthy" category because there is either enough evidence to suggest that they are not healthy or there is not enough evidence to indicate that they are healthy.

*Please note that I recommend primarily whole plant-based foods, even though I included animal products in category 2. Also, a food in the same category does not mean that it has an equivalent nutritive value.

Category four is difficult to limit to a rare indulgence, so Table 2 provides some alternatives. Alternative does not mean healthy; it just means that the food usually has less sugar, salt, and fat, and there may even be a nutritional benefit. Check the nutrition facts label and ingredients list for guidance on choosing the best options (see Chapter 13 on reading labels).

— TABLE 2 —
ALTERNATIVES TO "UNHEALTHY FOODS WITH NO REDEEMING QUALITIES" FROM TABLE 1

"UNHEALTHY FOOD CATEGORY"	BETTER ALTERNATIVE (DOES NOT MEAN HEALTHY)	HEALTHY (BEST) OPTION
Cookies (Chocolate/chip, sugar, shortbread, snickerdoodle, etc.)	Ginger snap cookies Coconut macaroons Oatmeal cookies Rice Krispies treats Granola bars Fig bars	Fruit Dark chocolate Oat bites Dates Dried figs Unsweetened dried fruit
Donuts	Bran muffin Granola bars Fig bars Milk chocolate	Fruit Dark chocolate Oat bites Dates
Cake (chocolate, yellow/vanilla, carrot, cheesecake, etc.)	Chocolate-covered berries or nuts Pudding Angel food cake or shortcake dessert cups with fruit and whipped cream	Fruit Dark chocolate
Potato/Tortilla Chips	Baked options Veggie/bean chips Rice cakes/snacks Green pea snacks	Carrot/celery sticks Cherry tomatoes Cucumber slices Roasted chickpeas/snacks Other veggies
Soda and Sugary Beverages (lemonade, sweet teas, etc.)	100% Juice	Water Unsweetened iced tea Sparkling water (without sugar or artificial sweeteners)
Macchiatos and Mochas	Latte	Coffee Tea
Ice Cream	Frozen fruit bars/pops Freezy/icy pops Some frozen yogurts Milk chocolate	Dark chocolate Homemade 100% fruit juice popsicles (See Chapter 5.)

"UNHEALTHY FOOD CATEGORY"	BETTER ALTERNATIVE *(DOES NOT MEAN HEALTHY)*	HEALTHY (BEST) OPTION
Pizza	Veggie pizza (See Chapter 8.) Cauliflower crust pizza Thin crust pizza	Eggplant pizza
Burgers	Veggie burgers (not including soy and plant-based meat alternatives)	Homemade black bean veggie burgers (See Chapter 8.)
Macaroni and Cheese	Mac n cheese with butternut squash puree	Mashed potatoes Sweet potato mash
Salad Dressings (ranch, blue cheese, Ceasar)	Italian dressing Honey mustard French dressing	Olive oil Lemon/lime juice Vinaigrettes
Cheese (cheddar, pepper jack, American and provolone)	Parmesan cheese Feta cheese Nutritional yeast	Fresh herbs and spices

*For meal suggestions mentioned in this chart, consider searching online for easy, affordable versions.

Here are some definitions that will be important for us to be on the same page about:

- ☑ Diet = what we eat daily (not a strict food regimen where foods are eliminated).
- ☑ Healthy foods = foods that contain the nutrients needed for optimal health and do no harm.
- ☑ Processed foods = foods that are mostly made from factory-made additives (like artificial colors, stabilizers, artificial sweeteners, and preservatives) and/or natural foods stripped of their nutrition (like sugar, flour, and oils). They also include hot dogs, sodas, shelf-stable cookies, etc.
  - Things to look out for with processed foods:
    1. The degree of processing. The further the product is from its natural state, the more processed it is and the worse for your health it is likely to be. Think potato chips versus potatoes. Potato chips are highly processed (or ultra-processed), while potatoes are not processed. Although some might argue that they are minimally processed.

2. How many chemicals and factory-made ingredients are in the item? Think rolled oats versus a store-bought granola bar. Rolled oats have fewer chemicals and other processed ingredients (and are less processed themselves) and, therefore, are better for optimal health.

Cream versus Oreo cookie filling is an interesting example. The cream is processed milk, whereas an Oreo cookie filling is an ultra-processed, factory-made item resembling cream. However, it does not contain milk, the main component of cream. Some of the older Oreo packages had the word 'creme' in place of cream on the package because it is not real cream. Neither product would be considered healthy per our definition, and both are processed, but one could be regarded as inordinately worse for our health than the other because of point number 1. The degree of processing and 2. The amount of chemicals and factory-made ingredients that are in the item. More on identifying healthy packaged foods in Chapter 13.

The "How to Prepare" Sections in Place of Recipes

Part of this book is designed to help you gain confidence in the kitchen. Therefore, instead of providing recipes with specific ingredient quantities and hard and fast rules, you will find the "How to Prepare" sections. These are suggestions for preparing meals and snacks. They provide multiple ingredient options for you to try. They serve to encourage tasting while preparing your food, increasing ingredient quantities as you go along based on your taste preferences. I will include quantities when I feel it is necessary for the base of the preparation instructions, but otherwise, I want you to feel empowered to trust yourself.

Small Changes Make a Big Difference

Throughout this book, I will focus on healthy foods as defined above. I want you to know that the ideal scenario is to eat only healthy food. However, that can be difficult for most of us. That is why many of my colleagues and I recommend working your way up to an 80:20 scenario. That is about 80% healthy and 20% whatever you want to eat. If you are starting out at 30:70, for example, work your way up to 35:65 and keep going. I know some people who go above 80% healthy, so don't limit yourself and go at a pace that works for you. Remember, small changes make a big difference no matter where you start.

Now let's begin with some savings, simple food preparation methods, and meal ideas.

PART 1

THE TOOLS

FOOD PREPARATION METHODS, MEALS, AND MORE

CHAPTER 1

EASY FOOD PREPARATION METHODS

If you feel overwhelmed by the thought of cooking or learning new techniques, this section is for you. While some of the meals in this book do not require any cooking, there are some simple cooking techniques that you can use to prepare affordable healthy meals. Before preparing healthy meals, let's look into what a healthy meal should consist of.

What Should a Healthy Meal Consist of?

You may have heard that a complete meal should include vegetables, protein, and a starch. However, there are no hard and fast rules for defining a meal. The most important thing is to get the nutrients you need daily, even if that means eating several snacks throughout the day instead of full meals.

There are several theories about how often we should eat meals. For example, fasting for 16 hours and eating everything in an 8-hour window (or some version of that) is one theory believed to reverse disease and help with weight management. Another theory is to eat 1-2 hours before and after drinking to allow your body to focus on digesting solids optimally. There is no right or wrong way to do it. The fact is that several people benefit from these different techniques.

Try different things and see what works for you; the most important thing is to get the nutrition you need for optimal health.

> Plant-based whole foods are almost always more affordable than animal products and processed plant-based foods.

Many of the starches we are used to eating (rice, pasta, bread, or other grains) pair nicely with traditional meals. They are filling and a good time but not necessary for optimal health. Since vegetables and healthy proteins have so many of the nutrients we need (including starches from things like beans and sweet potatoes), we will focus mostly on cooking techniques for vegetables and proteins.

Table 1.1 shows that focusing on healthy proteins and vegetables is very affordable. Healthy animal proteins can be affordable, but healthy plant-based proteins are the healthiest and, thank goodness, the most affordable.

— TABLE 1.1 —
COST OF "HEALTHY" MEALS THAT INCLUDE VEGETABLES AND PROTEINS WITH AND WITHOUT STARCHES

	COST OF A HEALTHY MEAL FOR A FAMILY OF FOUR			
	VEGETABLE + PLANT-BASED PROTEIN	VEGETABLE + PLANT-BASED PROTEIN + STARCH	VEGETABLE + ANIMAL PROTEIN	VEGETABLE + ANIMAL PROTEIN + STARCH
Vegetable (e.g., broccoli, sweet potato, spinach)	$3.00-$5.00	$3.00-$5.00	$3.00-$5.00	$3.00-$5.00
Protein (e.g., black bean burgers, tofu, or roasted chicken)	$2.00-$5.00	$2.00-$5.00	$7.00-$9.00	$7.00-$9.00
Starch (brown rice, quinoa)	–	$1.00-$4.00	–	$1.00-$4.00
Total Cost	$5.00-$10.00	$6.00-$14.00	$10.00-$14.00	$11.00-$18.00

All of the above are comparable to or cheaper than a fast-food meal for four which can cost upward of $20. Also, nutrient-rich meals are delicious and can take less time to prepare than going to a fast-food restaurant. Let's explore simple cooking techniques to create tasty, affordable, healthy meals.

Cooking Basics

Cooking can be fun. The following cooking techniques also happen to be healthy and easy. You can use each method in this chapter for multiple foods and never get bored. That is why I created a "Best Foods For" section for each cooking technique. If a food is not listed, that does not mean that it is not fair game. A few other things to note:

1. For some of these techniques, you will see "your cooking sweetener, milk, or sweetener of choice." Upcoming chapters have information on choosing the sweetener (chapter 14), milk (chapter 14), and oil (chapter 15) that works best for your budget and health.

    While healthier oils like avocado oil and sweeteners like raw honey are more expensive than things like vegetable oil and white sugar, you can get around that hefty price by using less, so you don't have to buy as much. The other workaround is to ask for them as gifts (and then use them sparingly).

    We've been conditioned to crave extra sweet and extra fatty foods, but tips throughout this book will help us appreciate naturally sweet and fatty foods so that we don't have to use them so much.

2. If you can get stainless-steel cooking pots and pans, do it. Ask for them as a gift even (more on that in chapter 2). They last forever and do not emit toxins into food like other materials, such as Teflon, non-stick, and aluminum. Cast iron is another safe option.

3. You will note that I do not mention beef or pork in any meals. Again, that is because we are focusing on healthy foods. But remember, just because it is not here does not mean it is

off-limits. No food is off-limits because we are going at our own pace and setting our own rules based on what we know and our current capacity.

4. If you choose to eat poultry, meat, or fish, there is a surefire way to determine when it is safe after cooking: Use a meat thermometer and make sure your food reaches a safe temperature. Thermometers start at around $7.00. Table 1.2 provides safe temperatures for a variety of foods.

— TABLE 1.2 —
THE UNITED STATES DEPARTMENT OF AGRICULTURE SAFE MINIMUM INTERNAL TEMPERATURES[3]

SAFE TEMPERATURES
"Cook all food to these minimum internal temperatures as measured with a food thermometer before removing food from the heat source. For reasons of personal preference, consumers may choose to cook food to higher temperatures."

PRODUCT	MINIMUM INTERNAL TEMPERATURE & REST TIME
Beef, Pork, Veal & Lamb Steaks, chops, roasts	145 °F (62.8 °C) and allow to rest for at least 3 minutes
Ground Meats	160 °F (71.1 °C)
Ground Poultry	165 °F
Ham, fresh or smoked (uncooked)	145 °F (62.8 °C) and allow to rest for at least 3 minutes
Fully Cooked Ham (to reheat)	Reheat cooked hams packaged in USDA-inspected plants to 140 °F (60 °C) and all others to 165 °F (73.9 °C).
All Poultry (breasts, whole bird, legs, thighs, wings, ground poultry, giblets, and stuffing)	165 °F (73.9 °C)
Eggs	160 °F (71.1 °C)
Fish & Shellfish	145 °F (62.8 °C)
Leftovers	165 °F (73.9 °C)
Casseroles	165 °F (73.9 °C)

Vegetables and Plant-Based Proteins

Vegetables and plant-based proteins don't need to be cooked to internal temperatures; just cook them to your desired texture.

If you eat them raw, it is essential to wash/scrub them thoroughly with water (a little vinegar or baking soda may also be used to clean them).

It is also important to avoid cross-contamination in the kitchen if you cook with meat. To do this, make sure your vegetables never touch raw meat. Use separate cutting boards and knives for each. Or chop up and clean vegetables first. If you use the sink, cutting board, knives, etc., for handling raw meat first, sanitize all surfaces with sanitizer, including hands, before working with the vegetables.

> The Food and Drug Administration allows meat manufacturers to sell meat to us even if it contains pathogens like bacteria! This is why it is so important to cook food to safe temperatures.

The healthiest way to eat fruit and non-starchy vegetables is raw. Whenever you add heat to vegetables, some element of the nutrition will be destroyed. That does not render the vegetable useless or unhealthy, just a little (in some cases a lot) less nutritious, but nutritious nonetheless. There are a few vegetables where adding heat is beneficial, as is the case with tomatoes and spinach. But in general, raw is best for optimal nutrition. One of the reasons salad is used as the standard for healthy eating is because it incorporates different colored raw vegetables and even fruits. The popular saying is that "an apple a day keeps the doctor away." You can replace the word "apple" with salad too.

A Few Cooking Notes

- ☑ Depending on the amount of food you want to cook, it only takes about 1-2 tablespoons of oil to coat it with oil.
- ☑ I recommend different times for specific cooking techniques. These are only guides. Cook your food to your desired texture, even if that means cooking it for shorter or longer periods.

- ☑ When cutting vegetables to cook, choose whatever shape you'd like (e.g., cubes, thin slices, thick slices, rectangles, etc.). Make the pieces the same size as much as possible so that they will cook more evenly.
- ☑ The instructions include ingredient measurements, but they are only recommendations. Switch them up to suit your needs and tastes.
    a. If you are cooking for one or four people, halve or double the ingredient quantities based on your needs.
- ☑ When it comes to spices, you'll want to adjust them to your tastes. Start conservatively (see Tables 1.3 and 1.4); you can almost always add spices at the end.

— TABLE 1.3 —
HOW MUCH SEASONING TO ADD TO A RECIPE TO START

DRIED SEASONING	HOW MUCH TO START WITH
Basil	½ tablespoon
Black Pepper	¼ teaspoon
Cayenne pepper	¼ teaspoon
Chili powder	½ tablespoon
Cumin	1 teaspoon
Garlic Powder	½ tablespoon
Onion Powder	½ tablespoon
Oregano	1 teaspoon
Red pepper flakes	¼ teaspoon
Rosemary	1 teaspoon
Salt	1 teaspoon
Seasoning salt	½ teaspoon
Smoked paprika	½ teaspoon
Thyme	1 teaspoon

— TABLE 1.4 —
POPULAR HERB/SPICE COMBINATIONS FOR COOKING

FLAVOR	HERBS/SPICE COMBINATIONS	MEAL EXAMPLES
Standard Savory	Salt, pepper, garlic powder, onion, powder and cayenne pepper	Beans, soups/stews, roasted veggies, stuffed bell peppers
Rustic Earthy	Salt, pepper, rosemary, thyme, sage	Roasted potatoes, roasted winter squashes (like butternut or acorn squashes), roasted chicken, butternut squash soup
Italian	Salt, pepper, basil, oregano, garlic, thyme, red pepper flakes	Tomato sauces for pizza, spaghetti, lasagna and other pasta dishes
Dill	Salt, pepper, dill	Potato salad, roasted potatoes, tuna salad, cucumber salad, yogurt-based dips, fish
Mediterranean	Salt, pepper, garlic, parsley, coriander, cumin	Lentil soups, lentil patties, roasted potatoes
Mexican	Salt, pepper, cumin, chili powder, garlic powder, onion powder, red pepper flakes, smoked paprika	Tacos, burritos, beans and rice
Asian	Salt, pepper, garlic, ginger, onion, (sesame oil)	Vegetable stir fry, sauces and chicken

Now, let us cook!

Roasting/Baking

Roasting and baking are very similar cooking methods. The biggest difference between the two is that baking is done at lower temperatures (300°F-375°F) and, therefore, is reserved for more delicate foods like fish. The instructions below for roasting and baking are the same except for the temperature difference.

MATERIALS NEEDED TO ROAST/BAKE

A sheet/roasting/baking pan

APPROXIMATE PREP AND COOK TIMES

Prep Time: 10-30 minutes
Cook Time: 20-50 minutes

HOW TO ROAST VEGETABLES

1. Preheat oven to 400°F-425°F.
2. Cut vegetables to your preferred shape and size (Make them the same size so they will cook evenly.).
3. Place the cut vegetables on a sheet pan.
4. Rub just enough oil to coat vegetables (about 1 tablespoon).
5. Add salt, pepper, and other seasonings (see tables 1.3 and 1.4).
6. Mix the veggies until they are coated with the oil and spices.
7. Space out vegetables evenly on the sheet pan.
8. Roast at 400°F-425°F for 5-15 minutes depending on the vegetable.
9. Flip after 10-15 minutes and put back in the oven for another 10-15 minutes.
10. Keep doing this until the vegetables are golden brown or your preferred texture.

BAKING FISH

1. Preheat oven to 375°F.
2. Place fish on a baking sheet.
3. Rub both sides of the fish with just enough oil to coat.
4. Add salt and pepper or other seasonings.
5. Roast for 5-10 minutes.

Food Safety Alert: Washing your meat increases your risk of spreading contaminants throughout your kitchen. You will kill whatever germs you wash away when you cook as long as you cook to the correct temperature (see Table 1.2). Washing meat is fine if you disinfect ALL surfaces (including the places where the water splashed). However, washing the meat is unnecessary if you cook it to safe temperatures.

BEST VEGETABLES FOR ROASTING

VEGETABLES	COST FOR 4 SERVINGS
Asparagus	$4.00
Beets	$3.00
Bell Peppers	$4.00
Broccoli	$3.00
Brussels Sprouts	$3.00
Carrots	$2.00
Cauliflower	$4.00
Eggplant	$4.00
Parsnips	$4.00
Potatoes (including French Fries)	$3.00
Sweet Potatoes	$4.00
Winter Squashes (butternut, acorn, etc.)	$3.00
Zucchini	$3.00

PROTEINS FOR ROASTING/BAKING

OTHER FOODS FOR ROASTING/BAKING	COST FOR 4 SERVINGS
Whole Chicken/Turkey	$8.00
Skinless Chicken/Turkey Breasts	$8.00
Chicken/Turkey Breast Wings	$10.00
Fish	$8.00

Using Air Fryers Instead of Baking/Roasting:

Air fryers are often used as an alternative to frying. Some of my clients/students use them for almost everything. Air fryers are convenient, sometimes faster, and typically a healthy way to prepare food. If you can get one, it is nice to have. However, they can be costly, take up a lot of counter space, and are unnecessary because you can achieve similar results by roasting or baking.

A Note About Baked Goods

Do you use oatmeal, zucchini, black beans, alternative flour, and gluten-free ingredients to make baked goods? I hate to break the news, but that does not necessarily make the baked goods healthy. Why? Because they still have added sugars, other sweeteners (sometimes even artificial), flours, and other processed ingredients.

They may be *healthier* versions of baked goods. So, yep, cookies made with half the sugar are better for you. The brownies made with black beans, zucchini, or oatmeal? Yep, better. So please, by all means, choose the healthier version; *it will make a difference.* The problem is that some of us tend to eat more because it is a healthier alternative. If you choose the healthier version, stick with one serving.

> Healthier versions of baked goods are a great way to make small changes that make a big difference. However, healthier does not mean that the food is healthy, so eat in moderation.

Healthy options include non-baked goods made with all-natural whole ingredients like dates, nuts, and oats. These are very nutrient-rich and good for optimal health. However, they can easily pack sugar and calories, so stick with portion sizes.

Sautéing

Sautéing is the process of cooking food quickly in a shallow pan at high heat with a small amount of fat. You don't have to be a good cook to sauté, but if you learn to sauté, you can cook endless delicious, affordable, convenient meals. Because sautéing requires high heat (therefore destroying some nutrients), some consider it as not the healthiest way to cook. And it's not; however, it is a better alternative to frying/deep frying. No batter is needed, and you only use one or two tablespoons of fat.

MATERIALS NEEDED TO SAUTÉ

A sauté pan

APPROXIMATE PREP AND COOK TIMES

Prep Time: 5-10 minutes
Cook Time: 5-20 minutes

SAUTÉING VEGETABLES

1. Chop vegetables in your favorite shape (Try to make them the same size.).
2. Heat the pan on medium-high heat.
3. Test the pan to ensure it is hot by adding a few drops of water. If the droplets evaporate right away, you are ready to go.
4. Add 1 tablespoon of oil.
5. Allow the oil to heat up (If your oil is smoking, then it has burned. Avoid burning by using cooking oil with a higher smoke point [See chapter 15].).
6. Add chopped vegetables to the pan with hot oil.
7. Add spices (Salt and pepper work well for any vegetable.).
8. Turn the vegetables over often so that they do not burn on either side (You may need to turn the heat down.).
9. Cook for 3-20 minutes (depending on the type of vegetable) until the vegetable is soft throughout.

Tip: To add extra flavor to any vegetable, sauté onions until they are soft, brown, and sweet using the above instructions. Then, add several finely chopped garlic cloves to the sautéed onion and cook until fragrant. Add your vegetables to this delicious mixture and cook to your desired consistency.

SAUTÉING CHICKEN/SEAFOOD AND VEGETABLES FOR THE SAME MEAL

1. Sauté your chicken/seafood first using the instructions for sautéing vegetables.
    a. You can season the chicken before putting it in the pan.
2. Remove protein when it has reached a safe temperature, and do not wash the pan. The temperature will be hot enough to kill any pathogens, so you do not need to wash in this instance.
3. Add a tablespoon of oil and cook the vegetables in the same pan (see instructions above).

*To save time, simultaneously cook the protein and veggies in separate pans. Sautéing your proteins first and then cooking the vegetables in the same pan will take longer, but the vegetables will have that flavor from the protein.

BEST VEGETABLES FOR SAUTÉING

VEGETABLE	COST FOR 4 SERVINGS
Asparagus	$4.00
Bell Peppers	$4.00
Broccoli	$3.00
Brussels Sprouts	$3.00
Cabbage	$2.00
Carrots	$2.00
Cauliflower	$3.00
Collard Greens	$3.00
Corn	$2.00
Kale	$2.00
Green Beans	$4.00
Green Peas	$4.00
Mushrooms	$3.00
Onions	$2.00
Snow Peas	$4.00
Spinach	$3.00
Zucchini	$3.00

PROTEIN	COST FOR 4 SERVINGS
Chicken Cutlets	$8.00
Fish Fillets	$9.00

Steaming

Steaming is the process of cooking food with steam from boiled water. Compared to sautéing, it better preserves the nutrients in vegetables and is a very healthy way to prepare vegetables and fish. You'd be surprised how easy steaming can be and how delicious the food will taste with just some salt and pepper. Steaming baskets are available for between $5.00 and $10.00 at most kitchenware stores. Try to stick with stainless-steel baskets to avoid chemicals leaching into your food.

> Vegetables and a protein can be a filling meal. You can add a starchy food, but it is not necessary.

MATERIALS NEEDED FOR STEAMING

A saucepan/pot
Steamer basket ($5.00-$10.00)

APPROXIMATE PREP AND COOK TIMES

Prep Time: 3-10 minutes
Cook Time: 3-10 minutes

HOW TO STEAM VEGETABLES

1. Bring a pot of water (4-5 inches) to a boil.
2. Chop or slice your vegetables into your desired shape (Make them the same size.).
3. Put the steaming basket on top of the pot with boiling water.
4. Put chopped/sliced vegetables in the basket.
5. Allow them to soften to your liking (about 3-10 minutes, depending on the vegetable).

6. Remove the basket from the pot and season with your favorite spices.
7. **Optional step:** Add oil or a little bit of butter; just be aware that certain fats are better for the heart than others and that fats, in general, add a significant number of calories. See Chapter 15 for more information on fats.
8. **Optional step:** Squeeze lemon or lime wedges over the vegetables after seasoning with spices.

***Note:** If you do not have a steamer basket, you can put 1-2 inches of water in a pan. Put the vegetables directly in the pan with the water and cover it until the vegetables are soft.

BEST VEGETABLES FOR STEAMING

FOOD	COST FOR 4-6 SERVINGS
Asparagus	$4.00
Bell Peppers	$3.00
Bok Choy	$4.00
Broccoli	$3.00
Brussels Sprouts	$3.00
Carrots	$2.00
Cauliflower	$3.00
Corn	$2.00
Onions	$3.00
Green Beans	$3.00
Green Peas	$2.00
Mushrooms	$2.00
Snow Peas	$4.00
Spinach	$4.00
Zucchini	$3.00

*Note: Fish can be steamed using the same technique (4-10 minutes). Lemon juice is a nice addition to fish after steaming.

Slow Cooking

If you don't have a slow cooker or crockpot, I encourage you to invest in one if you have the space and money. They are worth their weight in gold and work well even if you buy the most affordable one, which starts at about $25.00.

Throw several ingredients in a slow cooker/crockpot, set it in the morning, and allow it to cook your meal during the day. When you come home from work, dinner will be ready. A crockpot is fabulous for preparing vegetarian meals, especially meals with beans like bean and vegetable soups, spiced beans, and chili.

MATERIALS NEEDED FOR SLOW COOKING

A slow cooker/crockpot

APPROXIMATE PREP AND COOK TIMES

Prep Time: 10-20 minutes
Cook Time: 4-8 hours

HOW TO USE A CROCKPOT

1. Prepare your ingredients, including spices (see tables 1.3 and 1.4 for spice combinations).
2. Add your ingredients to the pot.
3. Put the lid on the pot and snap it close (check the instructions on your crockpot; some require that you don't snap the lid).
4. Set it to high or low, depending on what you are cooking and how long you want it to cook.
5. Allow the food to cook slowly until it is done. Typically, this takes 3-4 hours on the high setting and 7-8 hours on the low setting.
6. **Optional Step:** Top with fresh herbs, sour cream/Greek yogurt, avocado slices, or whatever complements your dish.

FOOD YOU CAN PREPARE IN A CROCKPOT

FOOD	COST FOR 4-6 SERVINGS
Beans	$3.00
Chili (vegetarian)*	$10.00
Lentils	$3.00
Soup (of any kind)	Varies
Stews (of any kind)	Varies
Collard Greens	$5.00
Whole Chicken	$7.00
Chicken Breast	$9.00

*You can cook ground beef/turkey chili in a crockpot; it just requires cooking the ground beef/turkey first and adds about $6.00.

— TABLE 1.5 —
SIMPLE VEGETARIAN CROCKPOT IDEAS FOR BEGINNERS

SLOW COOKER/CROCKPOT IDEAS			
DISH	SUGGESTED INGREDIENTS	SUGGESTED SPICES	SETTING AND COOK TIME
Vegetarian Chili	Kidney or black beans, crushed tomatoes, chopped onions, chopped green peppers, minced garlic, cubed sweet potatoes, 3-4 cups water or broth, 1-2 tablespoons of oil.	Salt, black pepper, garlic powder, chili powder, cumin, red pepper flakes	High for 3-4 hours or Low for 6-8 hours
Simple Savory Lentils	Green lentils, chopped onions, minced garlic, chopped carrots, cubed potatoes, tomato sauce, 3-4 cups water or broth, 1-2 tablespoons of oil.	Salt, black pepper	High for 3-4 hours or Low for 6-8 hours
Easy Beans	Any bean, chopped onions, minced garlic, 4 cups of water, 1-2 tablespoons of oil.	Salt, black pepper	High for 3-4 hours or Low for 6-8 hours

*There are several affordable crockpot recipes available online.

Pickling

Pickling is a way to extend the shelf-life of food using an acid, like vinegar. It is also a way to save some cash. Instead of throwing away your extra vegetables, you can pickle them. Pickled vegetables are good for topping dishes, sandwiches, or salads and are extremely nutritious because they help build healthy gut bacteria (more on this later). There are many ways to pickle, but we will do it the easy way: the quick pickle way.

MATERIALS NEEDED FOR QUICK PICKLING

Glass/mason jars with a tight seal and no rust

APPROXIMATE PREP AND SET TIMES

Prep Time: 5-10 minutes
Set Time: 1-24 hours

HOW TO PICKLE VEGETABLES

1. Chop your vegetables into slices/sticks/whatever shape your heart desires.
2. Pack your glass mason jar with the chopped vegetables.
3. Make the liquid mixture (also called brine):
   - ☑ 1½ cups water
   - ☑ 1 cup vinegar (white vinegar is best—look for 5% acidity on the bottle)
   - ☑ 2 teaspoons salt
   - ☑ **Optional:** Add fresh herbs like rosemary, thyme, dill, garlic, or spices like red pepper flakes
   - ☑ **Optional:** Boil the brine ingredients.
4. Add the brine to the vegetables until the jar is full. Make more brine if you don't have enough to fill the jar.
5. Seal the jar.
6. Allow to sit for 1 to 24 hours. The longer you wait, the better it tastes.

*Pickled vegetables last for weeks. If you like more of a punch, add more vinegar, but do not add less, as the proportions above are important for food preservation/safety reasons.

> If you have children, they will love chopping the veggies and putting them in the liquid! They will also be more likely to eat the product because they helped make it.

BEST FOODS FOR PICKLING

VEGETABLES	COST FOR 4 SERVINGS
Asparagus	$4.00
Beets	$3.00
Bell Peppers	$4.00
Cabbage	$3.00
Carrots	$2.00
Cauliflower	$4.00
Cucumbers	$3.00
Ginger	$2.00
Green Beans	$4.00
Jalapeno/Hot Peppers	$2.00
Parsnips	$4.00
Radishes	$4.00
Red Onions	$3.00
Winter Squashes (butternut, acorn, etc.)	$4.00

*You can pickle fruits like peaches and pears; just add sugar to your brine. You can even add spices like cinnamon, cloves, and ginger. Experiment with foods not mentioned here.

Cooking Beans and Other Legumes

I cannot emphasize enough how beneficial beans are to health. This is why I gave them their own section. There is no controversy around beans. Unless you have certain medical conditions, the only negative thing you might hear about beans is that they cause gas. Prepared the right way, they are delicious and versatile, and they are one of the most affordable foods on the planet at $2.00 for about 10 servings. Because they have protein and fiber, they fill you up quickly, which means that you are likely to eat less and save even more.

Beans provide:

- ☑ B vitamins, which help break down food and boost energy levels.

- ☑ Fiber, which builds a treasure trove of healthy, disease-fighting bacteria in the gut, helps the immune system function optimally, is good for cholesterol levels, and cleans the colon by promoting healthy bowel movements and weight management.
- ☑ Protein, which is good for muscles, energy, and weight management.
- ☑ Calcium, which is good for your bones, teeth, nervous system, and blood pressure.
- ☑ Antioxidants, which help fight cancer and other diseases.
- ☑ Iron, which is important for making and circulating blood ensuring that all body parts receive the nutrients they need for optimal health and energy levels.

Plenty of evidence suggests that eating beans regularly reduces the risk of cardiovascular disease, reduces inflammation, prevents/manages diabetes, and helps with weight control.[4] One study even found that a compound found in beans can inhibit cancer cell proliferation.[5]

There are so many bean varieties and ways to prepare beans that it's hard to find individuals who don't like them. Here are just a few popular beans:

- Black
- Black-eyed peas
- Cannellini
- Fava
- Great Northern
- Kidney
- Lima
- Pinto
- Navy
- Soy

Legumes

Beans are a part of the legume family. Legumes also include the following, which have many of the same benefits as beans:
- Chickpeas
- Lentils
- Split peas
- Peas

Making a concerted effort to eat legumes, even once or twice a week, instead of meat or poultry, can have tremendous health benefits. I know I said that you should choose what works for you, but I really want to encourage you to make this one work.

Canned or boxed beans are a very convenient and affordable way to eat beans. However, cooking dried beans is more affordable, even healthier, and more environmentally friendly.

What About Gas?

You can do some things to reduce the amount of gas you experience from beans. These techniques may not work for everyone, but some individuals find that they help.
1. Chew your food well (This has other health benefits as well, see chapter 18.).
2. Soak the beans overnight in water and salt.
3. Sprinkle a little baking soda when soaking the beans (You only need a little bit–too much might alter the taste of the beans.).
4. Eat beans regularly—some people find that they don't get gas if they eat beans regularly.

I purposely did not include taking gas-reducing enzymes like Beano because they are expensive and do not work for everyone, but they are a legitimate way to relieve some of the gas.

MATERIALS NEEDED FOR COOKING BEANS

A saucepan/pot

APPROXIMATE PREP AND COOK TIMES

Prep Time: 5-10 minutes (does not include the overnight soak)
Cook Time: 60 minutes (4-8 hours if using a slow cooker)

PREPARING DRIED BEANS

1. Follow the instructions on the package, which usually look something like this:
    a. **Optional Step:** Soak one 16-ounce bag of beans overnight in water and a pinch of salt. If cooking for fewer people, use ¼ or ½ the bag.
    b. Rinse and drain beans and add them to a pot with 4-6 cups of water.
    c. **Optional Step:** I like to add a little salt to the water at the beginning of the cooking process.
    d. Bring water to a boil.
    e. When water boils, turn the heat down to medium and cover.
    f. Allow beans to cook until tender throughout (usually about 40-60 minutes).
    g. **Optional Step:** Sauté onions and garlic and add to the cooked beans.

This technique works for most bean types. You can then use these beans for various meals. Freeze leftover beans for future meals by putting them in a sealed container. You can also use a food storage bag.

WAYS TO ENJOY BEANS*
Beans with rice and vegetables
Bean burritos/tacos*
Vegetarian chili*
Bean dips
Bean salads
Bean soups (15 bean soup, black bean soup, etc.)
Topping for a salad
Black bean burgers*
Vegetarian stuffed bell peppers*

WAYS TO ENJOY OTHER LEGUMES
Hummus (made with chickpeas)
Chickpeas instead of meatballs in spaghetti
Chickpea curry
Roasted chickpeas (add cayenne pepper or cinnamon)
Lentil soup*
Lentil patties

*See Chapter 8 for meal instructions or find recipes online.

If you have children, make it a game to see who can find the healthiest, most affordable, delicious, and easiest recipe. Then, let them make the recipe (or help with the recipe if they are too young to make it by themselves).

Use The Internet for Recipe Ideas

There are some meal preparation instructions in chapters 6–8 in this book that I'd like to encourage you to try. I also encourage you to look for easy, affordable, and delicious recipes online. I use YouTube and Instagram a lot for recipes. Be careful; all the recipes on these sites may be healthier alternatives, but they may not be healthy. If they contain things like agave, stevia, bread, pasta, flour, and ultra-processed vegan food products, lay low.

Food Prep Challenge

Cooking can be overwhelming, but these techniques don't have to be. Try this challenge to help you get started.

1. Next time you go grocery shopping, pick a vegetable that costs $4.00 or less and is enough for four people.
2. Choose one of the following techniques:
   a. Roasting
   b. Steaming
   c. Sautéing
   d. Pickling
3. Try preparing the vegetable by using the instructions above for your chosen technique.
4. Challenge a friend or family member to do the same and share the results.
5. The following week, try another technique with another food and another (or the same) friend/family member.

> Most vegan "dairy" products like butter, cheese, and mayo are highly processed and expensive. If you want to do good for the planet, go for it, however, there is not enough evidence to show that they are good for health. Limit or avoid them if you are trying to achieve optimal health.

Now that you have some affordable and easy cooking techniques, let's talk about more savings.

CHAPTER 2

FOOD SAVINGS PRO TIPS

After reading this book, you will find that healthy food often costs less than unhealthy food. On top of the savings from buying these nutritious foods, there are ways to save even more. Use some tips below to help you achieve your healthy food goals on a budget.

1. **Visit Your Local Food Pantry or Food Distribution Center**

   If you have never visited a food pantry near you, this might be the time to start. This is probably one of the most overlooked resources for individuals looking to save money on food. Non-profit organizations throughout the country distribute food at no cost to anyone who wants or needs food. You can save hundreds of dollars a year by using their services.

   > Visit www.feedingamerica.org to find your local food bank. Contact them and they will connect you with food pantries/food distribution centers near you.

   They often provide nutrient-rich foods you can use, like beans, rice, peanut butter, and even fresh produce. To find a food pantry near you:

   1. Visit Feeding America's ("the largest charity working to end hunger in the United States.") website at www.feedingamerica.org.

2. Click on the "Find a Food Bank" tab on the website.
3. Enter your zip code or state to find a nearby food bank.
4. Click on the name of your food bank. There are two things you can do from there:
    a. Find the food bank phone number on the website and call the food bank directly. They can find locations, dates, and times of food distributions near you.
    b. Look up food distributions directly on the food bank website.

*See Chapter 21 for more food resources available at no cost.

2. Just Drink Water

If you have a food craving, try drinking water and see if it helps curb your craving. If you have low energy levels and don't want to depend on caffeine and sugar to pick you up, try drinking water throughout the day. If you have skin problems, try drinking water in place of other drinks. The health benefits of drinking water are plenteous. It is the healthiest beverage to drink and is also the least expensive to buy.

> Juices, sodas, milk and other drinks can add $10.00-$20.00 a week for a family of four. Drinking *filtered* tap water instead adds about $2.00 a week.

The only drink we need for optimal health is water, not orange juice, milk, coffee (arguably), soda, iced tea, lemonade, or sports drinks (you can get all the electrolytes you need from food). If you want to save money, just drink water (See Chapter 5 for information on choosing the best quality water).

Drinking water can help you save in other areas, like skin care. I don't wear foundation or any other makeup, but people often compliment my skin and ask about my skincare routine (And I was diagnosed with eczema at one point!). I tell them I use a mild natural soap every morning, and before bed, I use an exfoliant once every few weeks (if I remember), I drink lots of water, and I eat lots of veggies. This adds up to about $5.00 a month on skincare, excluding water and food.

Drinking water helps with headaches, making you less likely to spend money on headache medicines. It helps with weight loss and all types of health ailments, so you don't have to spend as much on weight loss programs, medications, and doctor's visits. Water truly is an amazing, natural, and affordable resource.

3. **Plan Your Meals**

    The more we plan our meals, the more likely we are to save. Going to the grocery store without a plan may cause us to spend more than we want to on groceries. Here are some time-saving meal-planning tips:

    1. Try to keep the staples mentioned in Chapter 3 on hand. Local food pantries are a cost-effective way to keep your pantry filled with these staples.
    2. Check to see what you already have before going to the store and build meals around that.
    3. Always eat something before going to the grocery store—you will buy less because you won't be hungry while buying. Trust me on this one.
    4. Check the local listings for discounts/coupons and plan your meals around those deals.
    5. Purchase ingredients that you can use for multiple meals. Something like frozen corn can be used for soups, tacos, or salads (including bean salads). Onions can be used for almost anything, and the same goes for yellow potatoes, sweet potatoes, broccoli, and most veggies.

6. Ten minutes before going to the grocery store, jot down a few meal ideas for breakfast, lunch, dinner, and snacks.
7. Plan to eat leftovers. If we plan to eat leftovers, we only need two to three ideas for each meal. The food seems to always taste better on the second day anyway.

4. **Use Coupons Wisely**

   Do you buy stuff you don't really want because it is on sale? I want to let you know that that is not saving. That is wasting money. Clipping coupons can save money but do yourself a favor when couponing: Find things you will create meals with and eat. Otherwise, let those other coupons go.

5. **Shop for Fruits and Vegetables That Are Frozen**

   You might see berries in the grocery store in the wintertime and think, "Nah, that costs too much." If your budget allows for it, though, I say go ahead and spend the extra dollars; it's worth it. If not, go for the frozen berries instead. They are still very healthy and are a fraction of the cost of fresh berries. I buy both fresh and frozen. A 16-ounce bag of frozen blueberries or strawberries costs $3.00. The organic versions cost $4.00.

   > To determine if a particular fruit is in season, check the price. In the fall and winter, berries can cost up to $8.00 for four servings. If that is too steep, buy frozen berries instead. In the summer, those same berries can cost as little as $3.00-$4.00 for four servings.

6. **Shop for Fruits and Vegetables That Are in Season**

   The fresh berries may not be as affordable in the winter, but in the summer…it is on. You can find them for $3.00 or $4.00 for three to four servings. Foods grown near you in their peak season will almost always cost less than those not in season.

For example, summer is the season for tomatoes and peaches so they will cost a lot less where it is hottest near you.

Is Buying Organic Worth it?

Yes, it is. Organic does not mean that it is 100% free of pesticides, hormones, and antibiotics. It does mean that there are significantly less than conventionally grown (or non-organic) foods. I highly recommend buying organic for everything from produce to dairy if you can fit it into your budget.

Table 2.1 lists the produce with the most (the Dirty Dozen) and least (the Clean Fifteen) pesticides. This list is issued by the Environmental Working Group (more on them later). If you can't do all organic, choose the organic versions of the items from the Dirty Dozen list. If you can't do organic right now, that is ok too.

— TABLE 2.1. —
FRUITS AND VEGETABLES WITH THE MOST AND LEAST PESTICIDES

THE DIRTY DOZEN (Have the Most Pesticides)	THE CLEAN FIFTEEN (Have the Least Pesticides)
• Strawberries • Spinach • Kale, collard and mustard greens • Grapes • Peaches • Pears • Nectarines • Apples • Bell and hot peppers • Cherries • Green beans	• Avocados • Sweet corn • Pineapple • Onions • Papaya • Sweet peas (frozen) • Asparagus • Honeydew melon • Kiwi • Cabbage • Mushrooms • Mangoes • Sweet potatoes • Watermelon • Carrots

7. **Store Fruits and Vegetables so That They Last!**

   I used to store lemons on the countertop until someone told me that they last longer in the fridge. When I stored the lemons on the countertop, they would harden after a while.

> www.ask.usda.gov is a great resource if you want to know more about storing food!

When I stored them in the fridge, they did not get hard and lasted longer. Now I can buy the bulk bag of lemons (it's cheaper per lemon) and not worry about them getting too hard before I eat them.

Knowing the best way to store food can save a lot of money. The USDA has a website, https://ask.usda.gov, that answers all of your food storage and safety questions. Tables 2.2 and 2.3 provide storage information for several fruits and vegetables for your reference.

— TABLE 2.2 —
FRUIT STORAGE GUIDE (INFORMATION FROM SEATTLE PUBLIC UTILITIES WEBSITE)[6]

FRUIT	WHERE TO STORE IT	HOW TO STORE IT
Apple	Fridge	Separate from other produce.
Apricots	Ripen on counter, then store in fridge.	Store loose.
Avocado	Ripen on counter, then store in fridge.	Store loose.
Bananas	Counter	Store away from other fruits and vegetables.
Berries (any kind)	Fridge	Store in a shallow container lined with a dry towel; leave lid slightly cracked for air circulation. Wash only when ready to eat.
Cantaloupe	Ripen on counter, then store in fridge.	Store loose.
Cherries	Fridge	Store in a plastic bag or sealed container. Wash only when ready to eat.
Grapes	Fridge	Store in a sealed container. Wash only prior to eating.
Grapefruit	Fridge-crisper drawer	Store loose.
Honeydew melon	Ripen on counter, then store in fridge.	Store loose.
Kiwi	Ripen on counter, then store in fridge.	Store loose.
Lemon	Fridge-crisper drawer	Store loose.
Lime	Fridge-crisper drawer	Store loose.
Lychee	Counter	Store loose.
Mandarin	Counter	Store loose.

FRUIT	WHERE TO STORE IT	HOW TO STORE IT
Mango	Ripen on counter, then store in fridge.	Store loose.
Nectarine	Ripen on counter, then store in fridge.	Store loose.
Orange	Fridge-crisper drawer	Store loose.
Papaya	Counter	Store loose.
Peach	Ripen on counter, then store in fridge.	Store loose.
Pear	Ripen on counter, then store in fridge.	Store loose.
Pineapple	Ripen on counter, then store in fridge.	Store loose.
Plum	Ripen on counter, then store in fridge.	Store loose.
Pomegranate	Fridge	Store loose.
Raspberries	Fridge	Store in a shallow container lined with a dry towel; leave lid slightly cracked for air circulation. Wash only when ready to eat.
Soursop	Counter	Store loose.
Starfruit	Counter	Store loose.
Strawberry	Fridge	Store in a shallow container lined with a dry towel; leave lid slightly cracked. Wash only when ready to eat.
Tangerine	Counter	Store loose.
Watermelon	Ripen on counter, then store in fridge.	Store loose.

— TABLE 2.3 —
VEGETABLE STORAGE GUIDE
(INFORMATION FROM SEATTLE PUBLIC UTILITIES)[7]

VEGETABLE	WHERE TO STORE IT	HOW TO STORE IT
Arugula	Fridge	Remove bands and ties. Store in a sealed container lined with a damp towel.
Asparagus	Fridge	Remove bands and ties. Store upright in a glass of water with a plastic bag over the top.
Beets	Fridge	Store in a sealed container with a dry towel. Store green tops separately (see "Leafy Greens").
Bell Peppers	Fridge-crisper drawer	Store loose
Bok Choy	Fridge	Remove bands and ties. Store in a sealed container lined with a damp towel.

VEGETABLE	WHERE TO STORE IT	HOW TO STORE IT
Broccoli, Broccolini	Fridge-crisper drawer	Wrap in a damp towel.
Broccoli Rabe	Fridge	Remove bands and ties. Store in a sealed container lined with a damp towel.
Brussel Sprouts	Fridge-crisper drawer	Store in a sealed container.
Cabbage	Fridge-crisper drawer	Store loose
Carrots	Carrots	Store in a sealed container with a dry towel. Store green tops separately (see "Leafy Greens").
Cauliflower	Fridge-crisper drawer	Store in a plastic bag or sealed container.
Celery	Fridge	Store in a sealed container.
Chard	Fridge	Remove bands and ties. Store in a sealed container lined with a damp towel.
Collard Greens	Fridge	Remove bands and ties. Store in a sealed container lined with a damp towel.
Corn	Fridge	Store loose.
Cucumbers	Fridge-crisper drawers	Store loose.
Eggplant	Fridge-crisper drawers	Store loose.
Green Beans	Fridge	Store in a plastic bag or sealed container.
Green Onions	Fridge	Wrap in a damp towel.
Herbs, leafy (Examples: cilantro, parsley)	Fridge	Remove bands and ties. Trim stems and store upright in a glass of water.
Herbs, woody (Examples: rosemary, sage)	Fridge	Remove bands and ties. Wrap in a damp towel and store in a sealed container.
Kale	Fridge	Remove bands and ties. Store in a sealed container lined with a damp towel.
Leafy Greens	Fridge	Remove bands and ties. Store in a sealed container lined with a damp towel.
Lettuce	Fridge	Remove bands and ties. Store in a sealed container lined with a damp towel.
Mushrooms	Fridge	Store in a paper bag.
Okra	Fridge	Store in a paper bag.
Onions	Cupboard/Pantry	Store loose or in a mesh bag separate from potatoes.
Parsnips and Turnips	Fridge	Store in a sealed container with a dry towel. Store green tops separately (see "Leafy Greens").
Squash (acorn, butternut, winter)	Cupboard/pantry	Store loose.

VEGETABLE	WHERE TO STORE IT	HOW TO STORE IT
Squash (zucchini, summer)	Fridge	Wrap whole or cut ends in a damp towel.
Tomatoes	Ripen on counter, then store in fridge.	Store out of direct sunlight.

8. **Check Unit Prices**

   Have you ever stood in the grocery store trying to determine if buying a larger or smaller product is cheaper? Well, stand around and do math no more. In general, it is cheaper per serving to purchase the larger size. But to be sure, look at the unit cost listed on the shelf where the product is found.

   The unit cost is the cost per unit of a particular item. They are found on the shelf next to the retail price. In Figure 1, the unit is one ounce. The cost per ounce is 16.7 cents for the smaller bottle and 13.6 cents for the larger bottle. This means that the larger item costs 3.1 cents less per ounce than the smaller bottle. Some of us may not be in a position to purchase the larger product, and that is ok; just be aware of this for when you will be in that position.

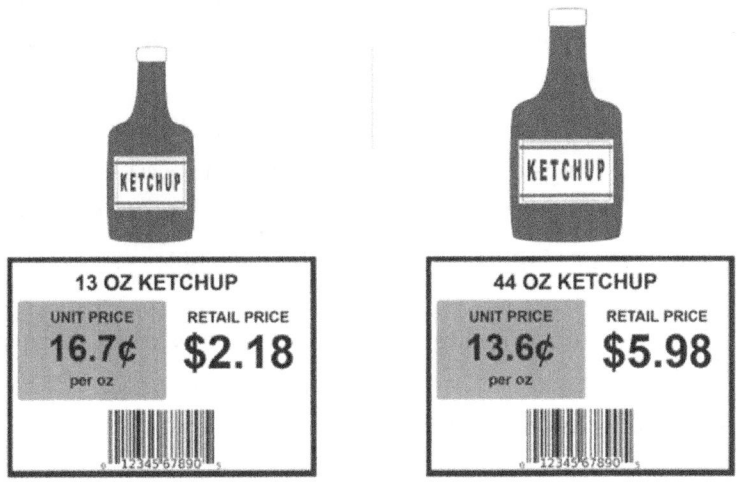

Figure 2. Comparing the unit price of a 13-ounce bottle of ketchup to a 44-ounce bottle of ketchup. [8]

We tend to eat bigger portions when we have more, making the savings null and void. If you buy the bulk item, try to stick with the serving size suggestions on the package. This is another way that serving sizes help us save money.

9. **Join a Warehouse Club**

   When I was younger, my mother gave my cousin money to buy a few grocery items from the grocery store or my cousin's warehouse club. These clubs have grocery items (and more) that you can buy in bulk. I mean really bulk. This means that per unit (see number 8), she was probably saving a lot of money. These clubs charge a membership fee somewhere between $60.00-$70.00 depending on the warehouse. They are also far away if you live in an urban or rural area. So, finding someone who already has a membership and goes regularly is a great option for savings.

   > Get together with your friends/family to buy a membership (usually about $60 a year). Take a trip together once a month to stock up on what you need.

   You can also purchase a membership as a group (everybody pays $15.00) and have someone do the runs to get the food items (or you can go together).

   Warehouses like Costco, Sam's, and BJ's are great for long-term savings if you can get past the membership fees and the bulk prices. For more savings, remember to stick to the serving size recommendations on the package.

The most nutritious items that you can buy from these warehouses are:
- Fresh produce
- Beans
- Lentils
- Nuts

- Frozen fruit and vegetables
- Dried fruit (preferably with no added sugar)
- Jarred fruits (Make sure it is in 100% juice, not syrup.)
- Jarred vegetables (like olives and pickles)
- Applesauce with no added sugar
- Peanut butter
- Spices
- Mustard
- Honey
- Vinegar
- Oatmeal
- Rice
- Greek yogurt
- Tea
- Coffee
- 100% juices
- Low-sodium vegetarian soups
- Popcorn

The healthiest items for meat eaters are:
- Frozen salmon
- Frozen chicken breast/chicken cutlets
- Tuna fish

These warehouses have several frozen entrées and sides. Use the nutrition facts label to choose the healthiest options (See chapter 13 for more information on using the nutrition facts label.). I highly recommend sticking with the vegetarian options as much as possible.

If you have a hard time resisting the urge to buy big bags of chips, bulk candies, muffins the size of your head, etc., make a list and try to stick to it. If you buy something you hadn't planned on buying, that is okay; don't beat yourself up. Just go with it.

10. **Take Advantage of Bargain/Dollar Store Deals**
    Some bargain/dollar stores have healthy options. The bargain/dollar store near me has the following options for $1.25:
    - Roasted peanuts
    - Skinny Pop popcorn
    - Rice
    - Beans
    - 100% whole wheat bread that costs the same as white bread (As you know, I am not a big proponent of bread, but if you're gonna do it, 100% whole grain is the best option for health.).
    - Applesauce (with no added sugar)
    - Spices
    - Vinegar
    - Coconut flakes
    - Hot sauce (with just peppers and salt)
    - Tostadas

11. **Buy Generic Brands**
    Don't let the brand name and fancy advertising fool you. In terms of quality, generic brands can be just as good as brand names. They even taste the same in many cases. Sometimes the generic tastes better.

    If the children/spouse won't eat it unless it has a specific brand name, put the generic brand contents in the box of the brand name. They won't know the difference. I can't tell you how many funny stories I heard about one spouse (or parent) switching the box without the other spouse and children noticing the difference.

12. **Purchase Collard Greens or Kale**
    Surprisingly, two of the most nutritious and filling foods in the entire supermarket are also two of the least expensive:

collard greens and kale. One bunch of kale or collard greens costs $2.49 year-round, even in today's market. They are filled with fiber and nutrition that is good for your vision, heart, blood sugar, weight, and even your brain. Here are just a few things you can do/make with collard greens or kale:

- Fantastic side dishes
- Salads
- Add them to soups and pastas
- Use the large leaves instead of bread for sandwiches
- Juice them

If you are interested in gardening, I highly recommend growing these two yourself (see Chapter 21 for more on gardening). They require little effort and grow easily, and every time you harvest them, they grow back within weeks. If you grow multiple plants, you can have them regularly when in season at no extra cost to you.

13. Make Open-Faced Sandwiches

An open-faced sandwich is just a sandwich with one slice of bread instead of two. It saves money and decreases bread and calorie intake.

Allow me to put a plug in for rice cakes instead of bread for certain sandwiches (like tuna or peanut butter). The Quaker Oats company has a rice cake with only one ingredient: brown rice, and it is delicious—believe me. Also, when I have my rare craving for bagels and cream cheese, I use rice cakes instead of bagels. They taste better than bagels with cream cheese (hard to believe, but trust me), and I save money at $4.00 for 14 cakes. Also, at 35 calories a serving, I save about 200 calories. I also eat them plain sometimes as a crunchy snack instead of chips.

Also, recall that you can use large leafy green leaves as a wrap instead of bread.

14. **Use Every Part of Your Food**

Some parts of vegetables that we throw away are edible. Eating these parts means more nutrition and fiber for you. It also means that you and your family will fill up faster and eat less, so you don't have to buy as much.

Here are some tips for using all parts of your vegetables:
1. Chop collard greens, kale, and broccoli stems really small and add them to salad—this adds a delicious crunch and filling fiber.
2. Make your own vegetable or chicken broth.
    a. <u>To Make Homemade Vegetable Broth:</u>
        i. After you finish chopping veggies for a recipe, put the scraps in boiling water and allow them to cook for 5-10 minutes. Use less water for a stronger-flavored broth.
        ii. Allow the water and veggies to cool off.
        iii. Strain the water and put it in a glass jar.
        iv. Store it in the fridge until you are ready to make your next recipe that requires broth. It is safe to eat for up to 3-4 days. You can also freeze it, and it will last for 2-3 months. Compost the leftover vegetables.
    b. <u>To Make Homemade Chicken Broth:</u>
        i. Add the parts of the chicken you did not eat (skin, bones, and all) to boiling water and cook for 5-10 minutes. Use less water for a stronger-flavored broth.
        ii. You can add herbs and spices, but the chicken alone is enough.
        iii. Strain the broth and store the savory liquid in the fridge. You can use it for up to 3-4 days. You can also freeze the broth. Compost the unused parts of the chicken.

3. Make citrus zest. Scrape the rinds of citrus fruits (lemon, lime, oranges, etc.) with a zester to flavor food. Zesters cost $5.00-$10.00 and add amazing flavor. Here are some things you can do with citrus zest:
    a. Add to homemade salad dressing (see Chapter 7).
    b. Add to fruit sauces like berry or pear sauce (see below).
    c. Top fruit and whipped cream.
    d. Top pasta dishes.
    e. Top potato wedges.
4. Use overripe fruit. You can do something with that fruit that is about to go bad.
    a. If you have a blender, make a smoothie with the overripe fruit (see Chapter 5).
    b. Make a fruit sauce you can add to plain yogurt or use instead of syrup. To make the fruit sauce (or compote):
        i. Clean and chop up the fruit (if necessary).
        ii. Throw it in a saucepan with enough water to cover the fruit.
        iii. Allow the fruit to soften, and mash it until it is the texture you like.
        iv. **Optional Step:** Add citrus fruit zest or spices like cinnamon or fresh/ground ginger.
5. Use overripe veggies. You can also do something with those overripe veggies that are about to go bad.
    a. Make an easy vegetable soup. Here's how:
        1. Sauté chopped onions and garlic until they are soft and fragrant.

2. Add a few cups of water or broth and any chopped vegetables you want to use before they go bad to the onions and garlic.
3. Add salt, pepper, thyme, rosemary, parsley, or red pepper flakes. Salt and pepper are fine by themselves.
4. Cook until the vegetables are soft and the flavors meld together.
5. Add cooked chickpeas, beans, pasta, barley, or rice (whatever you have on hand) and allow the soup to simmer for 10 more minutes.

b. Juice the veggies if you have a juicer.
1. If you grow your own food, compost the scraps, and make your own soil (see chapter 21).

15. **Use the USDA Food Keeper Website/App**

    Have you ever thrown away food because you weren't sure if it was still good? If you have, you might have wasted that food and your money.

    The United States Department of Agriculture (USDA) has an app that provides food storage times before the food is unsafe to eat. It also provides tips for storing foods to keep them fresh longer. The app includes produce (vegetables and fruits), meat, poultry, eggs, frozen foods, vegetarian proteins, lemon juice, leftovers, and more.

    > The USDA Food Keeper Website provides food storage times and storage tips that can save money.

    1. Visit the website https://www.foodsafety.gov/keep-food-safe/foodkeeper-app (or do a web search for the USDA Food Keeper).
    2. Click the search tab.

3. In the search box, type the item you are looking for and find the item.

16. **Know What Those "Sell by" and "Best by" Dates Mean**
The dates on food are not food safety dates; they are food quality dates. That means the food is safe to eat after that date; it's just not peak quality. If you have some canned products, rice, eggs, and yogurt, they may still be safe to eat after the best-by/use-by date. Use the USDA Food Keeper site (see number 15) to help determine if your food is still safe to eat.

CAUTION: If the food smells bad and you can see that it has gone bad, throw it away no matter the date.

17. **Pay Attention to Serving Sizes and Use Measuring Cups**
This may seem like an unusual way to save money, but it is savings at its best. Every packaged food has a recommended serving size on the nutrition facts label. We tend to ignore that recommendation and pile food on with reckless abandon. For example, the next time you eat cereal, do this:
    1. Pull out two bowls.
    2. Pour the cereal as you normally would in one bowl.
    3. In the other bowl, before pouring the cereal, look up the serving size and measure it using a measuring cup.
    4. Compare the two bowls.

Following the serving size recommendations will make your food last much longer, and you won't have to buy as much.

18. **Revolutionize Gift Giving**
Instead of lotions, potions, and trinkets you will never use, make a pact with certain friends/family to give food/food-related gifts instead. How about:
    - A nice bottle of olive, coconut, or avocado oil

- Apple cider/balsamic vinegar
- Some nuts (I sometimes give large bags of pecans and walnuts as gifts)
- A spice pack
- A nice glass food storage container set
- A water filter (see Chapter 4)
- A glass or stainless-steel water bottle
- A grocery store gift card
- A customized staple foods gift basket with a pretty bow
- A membership to a warehouse club
- A lemon zester or nice measuring cups
- A slow cooker/crockpot

I have given and received gifts like this often and am always excited when I receive them. The person I give the gift to is also usually happy (at least they seem to be).

19. Can I Encourage You to Grow Herbs?

Fresh herbs typically cost $3.00 and are usually enough for one meal. An herb plant might cost the same amount but will last multiple meals for months. See Chapter 21 for gardening tips and how to maintain herb plants indoors. Herbs are easy to grow and keep. They add a burst of flavor that you often can't get from dried spices and pack a powerful nutrient punch. Children love to take care of and watch the plants grow. They also love to use the food that they grew themselves.

> Lots of children love to take care of and watch plants grow. Get them started with growing herbs. They will also want to eat them too!

20. Only Cook What You Need.

I am known for having a half-filled bag of lentils and beans sitting in the pantry with a tight rubber band around it. That is because I try only to cook what I need. You can save or freeze the leftovers if you cook too much, which saves a lot of time. However, sometimes, it's fine not to cook it all in the first place. If you cook what you need, the next time you go grocery shopping, that is one less thing you will have to worry about/spend money on.

With these food-saving tips, you can save a lot of money. I mentioned that you can save money by getting food from a food pantry or food distribution near you. Let us now look at some standard staple foods often found at these food distributions to ensure you always have the basics on hand to make a meal.

CHAPTER 3

STAPLE FOODS TO HAVE ON HAND

Certain foods are worth their weight in gold in the kitchen. They are affordable, can be used for multiple meals and snacks, and often can be stored for weeks or months without going bad. Many of my clients/students like to stock up on these staples so they don't have to worry about purchasing them every time they go grocery shopping. Tables 3.1, 3.2, and 3.3 list healthy staple foods to have on hand.

— TABLE 3.1 —
HEALTHY SHELF-STABLE STAPLE FOODS

SHELF-STABLE FOODS	
Beans	Oil
Brown rice	Peanut butter
Corn tortillas	Quinoa
Diced tomatoes	Salsa
Dried fruit	Vinegar
Lentils	100% Whole wheat/grain crackers
Marinara/tomato pasta sauce	100% Whole wheat/lentil/bean pasta
Mustard and other condiments	Vegetable broth*
Nuts	Spices
Oatmeal	

*Or make your own (see Chapter 2).

How to Stock up on Staples

- ☑ Use coupons.
- ☑ Buy the larger size.
- ☑ Shop at warehouses/clubs.
- ☑ Use food pantries or food distributions near you.
- ☑ Use government assistance programs (see Chapter 21).
- ☑ Stock up on spices slowly.

There is nothing like the right spice for the right dish. Below is a list of spices to grab if you can. You can build up your collection gradually or ask for a spice set for your birthday or holiday gift. Spices are safe to eat for years after purchase, so don't worry about them going bad. However, you will want to use them faster for the most potent flavor.

— TABLE 3.2 —
SPICE RECOMMENDATIONS

SPICES TO HAVE ON HAND		SPICES NICE TO HAVE ON HAND
Black pepper	Nutmeg	Bay leaves
Cayenne pepper	Onion powder	Cloves
Chili powder	Oregano	Coriander
Cinnamon	Red pepper flakes	Rosemary
Cumin	Salt	Smoked paprika
Garlic powder	Turmeric	Thyme
Ground ginger		

Perishable Foods

Whenever I see a three-pound bag of onions on sale for $1.49, I grab two or three bags because I know they will last me for weeks. Table 3.3 lists healthy perishable foods that last two to four weeks and cost no more than $4.00-$5.00. Have these on hand for delicious, affordable meals.

— TABLE 3.3 —
PERISHABLE FOOD RECOMMENDATIONS

PRODUCE TO HAVE ON HAND	
Potatoes	Carrots
Sweet potatoes	Fresh garlic
Onions (yellow, white or red)	Winter squashes (butternut, acorn, etc.)

Build Your Staples Shelf Slowly

This chapter contains several recommendations, which is why I want to remind you that you do not need everything on these lists. Build your staples shelf/pantry slowly if you have to, and refill it regularly. Go item by item, gift by gift, and food pantry by food pantry.

Now that we have discussed our staples, let's discuss how to prepare them. But first, we have to drink, don't we?

CHAPTER 4

DRINKS

I once ordered a mocktail (that is, a cocktail without alcohol) while out to dinner with my husband. I normally order water, but this was a splurge day, and a virgin mojito was on my mind. The drink turned out to be delicious. It did not have alcohol, so I figured it would cost about the same price as some of the other non-alcoholic beverages. Maybe a little more because there's some work involved in making it. When the bill came, it said that my virgin mojito cost twelve dollars. You read that right—twelve dollars for some sparkling water, syrup, a lime wedge, and a sprig of mint. And it's not even healthy. I mean, the nerve! But they charge that amount because people will pay for it. And we pay for it because we love our drinks.

As You Keep Reading, Keep These Things in Mind:
1. Be encouraged.
2. Be open to trying new things.
3. You don't have to change everything overnight or anything at all. The point of this book is to provide awareness so that you can make informed decisions that fit your situation.
4. You do not have to stop drinking/eating your favorites.
5. RELAX, and take things step by step!

This chapter presents a list of delicious, healthy, affordable drink options that you will love but not at the $12.00 price point. Heck, it won't even be at the $3.00 per ½ gallon price point like some soda pops and other sugary beverages.

This book is about achieving optimal health on a budget, so we will get into the weeds a little regarding chemicals in our food and drinks and discuss what we can do to reduce these chemicals and their harmful effects. Often, it is less expensive to avoid these chemicals than to eat/drink them. Let's start with some healthy drink options.

Water

Clean water is the healthiest beverage anywhere at any time. There are significant health benefits to drinking other beverages like tea, but there is nothing like water. Water makes up 60%-70% of our body and is used for almost every reaction that our bodies need to survive. Here are just a few of the thousands of benefits of drinking water regularly:

1. Better energy levels (Energy drinks and coffee cost more than water and don't work as well over the long term.)
2. Weight management (If only I had a dollar for every time someone told me they lost weight by switching to water only.)
3. Helps regulate blood pressure
4. Helps to manage diabetes
5. Prevents/reduces headache pain
6. Prevents/reduces arthritis pain and inflammation
7. Clearer skin
8. Prevents/helps relieve constipation
9. Water helps the kidneys to flush toxins out of the body better and helps the kidneys function better
10. Helps to prevent bladder infections

11. It does a lot more, and it costs less than most unhealthy beverages (see Table 4.1)

— TABLE 4.1 —
PRICE COMPARISON BETWEEN WATER AND SODA

	BOTTLED WATER	SODA/POP
Average price per ½ gallon	$0.75 ($1.50/gallon)	$2.00
Average price per 12 bottles (bought in bulk)	$2.00 ($0.17 per 16-oz. bottle)	$6.00 ($0.50 per 16.9-oz. bottle)

*A good water filter will provide clean water for 3-6 months for less than $25.00 (see next section).

We live in a world where significant contamination reaches our food and water supply. To optimize our health, here are some tips on drinking the safest water possible.

Water Filters

PFAS (or Per—and Polyfluoroalkyl Substances) and lead are contaminants that find their way into our tap water. The federal government sets what it calls "maximum contaminant levels" for several of these chemicals. In other words, cities and states are not to exceed these limits.

PFAS, also called forever chemicals, are not found in nature and don't break down in the environment. They build up once they enter the human body through our water and food supply. This buildup may be linked to certain cancers and may suppress our immune systems, making us more susceptible to viruses like COVID.[9]

Using a water filter is something we can do to reduce our intake of forever chemicals. There are also other benefits to using a water filter:
- The water tastes better.
- It costs less over the long term.
- It's better for the environment than bottled water.

- It is healthier (no/reduced plastic, PFAS, lead, or other chemicals in the water).
- You can request one for a birthday/holiday/whatever you celebrate present.

This is why I recommend using a water filter instead of bottled water or drinking water directly from the tap.

Best Affordable Water Filter

The Environmental Working Group (EWG) is a non-profit community made up of people who work to protect public health. They tested several filters for these forever chemicals and found that the ZeroWater filter eliminates 100% of PFAS and is recommended for best results. At the writing of this book, the ZeroWater pitcher starts at $22.00 for a 7-cup pitcher that lasts 3-4 months on one filter. The replacement filters are about $17, which is about $5.00 a month.

There are other affordable water filters found on the shelves of grocery and big box stores that filter out some of these forever chemicals; they are effective also, just may not be as effective as the ZeroWater filter.

A Note About Water Bottled in Plastic

Bottled water (and other beverages) often contains forever chemicals. Water and other beverages in plastic bottles have forever chemicals plus small plastic particles (micro/nano plastics) that present additional threats to our health. The FDA regulates bottled beverage companies but allows them to sell us contaminated drinks. It just sets maximum levels for the contaminants.[10]

I recommend drinking filtered tap water from glass cups or bottles instead of bottled in plastic. Filters are the healthier, more affordable, and environmentally friendly option. Plastic bottles that are not recycled have a final destination, which may include the ocean or landfills. When the plastic reaches its destination, it breaks down again into micro/nano plastics that wind up in our water and food, giving us double the dose of plastic.

If that weren't enough reason to reduce plastic, we are running out of space to put it. Recycling helps some (so please recycle), but not nearly enough to contain the problem. Buy a stainless-steel water bottle and fill it with filtered water for when you are on the go. You will save a lot of money and improve your health.

> Try to avoid drinking from plastic (even reusable water bottles). If you do drink from them, do not leave plastic bottled drinks in the heat (especially in a hot car). More plastic will melt and leach into the drink. Use glass or stainless-steel water bottles instead.

About Glass Bottles

If you can find water bottled in glass, it truly is better for your health. Even though glass presents its own set of environmental problems, unlike plastic, glass can be reused and recycled safely and indefinitely. Unfortunately, it is more expensive and usually comes in smaller portions. Glass and stainless-steel water bottles are safe to use. Fill them with filtered water for when you are on the go.

— TABLE 4.2 —
DRINKING WATER SAFETY SUMMARY

WATER TYPE	PROS	CONS
Tap Water	• No artificial or ultra-processed ingredients like sugar, high fructose corn syrup, and artificial sweeteners added	• Has high mineral levels and forever chemicals that may cause developmental/health problems over time
Water in Plastic Bottles	• No artificial or ultra-processed ingredients, such as sugar, high fructose corn syrup, and artificial sweeteners added • Most filter out some of the chemicals found in tap water (however, many are still contaminated)	• Many contain forever chemicals that may cause developmental/health problems over time • Plastic leaches into the water (especially if left in heat), which may cause developmental/health problems over time • Breaks down into micro/nano plastics that leach into water and food systems • Creates landfill and ocean waste

WATER TYPE	PROS	CONS
Water in Glass Bottles	• No artificial or ultra-processed ingredients like sugar, high fructose corn syrup, and artificial sweeteners added • Most filter out some of the chemicals found in tap water • No plastic leaching into the water • Safe to reuse and recycle	• Many contain forever chemicals that may cause developmental/health problems over time • More expensive • Not as accessible • Creates landfill and ocean waste
Water Filter	• No artificial or ultra-processed ingredients like sugar, high fructose corn syrup, and artificial sweeteners added • Most filter out the chemicals found in tap water • No plastics leaching into the water • Safe to reuse • Best for the environment • THE BEST OPTION BY FAR!	• May not filter 100% of forever chemicals depending on the brand

Below are more healthy and affordable drink suggestions.

Homemade Infused Water
$1.00 for the fruit/herb for multiple servings

Because sugary beverages, sports/energy drinks, and other drinks are made with water (often not filtered), they, too, may contain forever chemicals and nanoplastics (from plastic bottles). To add insult to injury, they also contain sugars, artificial colors, and other substances in large quantities that evidence suggests are harmful to our health.

We usually don't have sugary beverages in our fridge/pantry, so when we have guests, we offer filtered or bottled water depending on their preference. One drink that I usually have on hand during the summer is cold fresh mint water. We have a water filter, and I grow mint on the deck, so it costs nothing to make. Yet, the reaction from my guests is often utter surprise and delight at how refreshing and delicious the water tastes. Sometimes, I even send them home with sprigs of mint so they can make their own.

Mint water is my favorite infused water, but many herb/fruit options exist. It is delicious, thirst-quenching, adds nutrients to the water, and is more affordable than most unhealthy beverages. Simply drop herb sprigs (or fruit slices if you want to use fruit) into the water and allow it to sit overnight in the fridge. Popular infused waters are:
- Mint
- Cucumber
- Lemon
- Lime

You can also experiment with your favorite flavors. Strawberries, fresh basil, watermelon, orange, and grapefruit are all fair game.

Seltzer Water
$1.00 for a 16-ounce bottle

We know the downfalls of drinking from plastic bottles, but let's be real: most of us drink from plastic occasionally. When we do, it is more important to choose the healthiest drinks possible. Aside from water, the healthiest options are bottled flavored waters (mentioned in the previous section) and seltzer waters *without* artificial/sweeteners. The healthiest seltzer options have no more than two ingredients on the ingredients list: carbonated water and natural flavors. Avoid artificial sweeteners (See Chapter 13 for more on identifying artificial sweeteners.).

> There are multiple flavored waters on the market with water, natural flavors and nothing else. They are usually less expensive than the sodas and other unhealthy drinks.

Seltzer Water Brands That I Recommend

These brands usually have carbonated water and natural flavors only. Always check the ingredient lists to make sure.
- Polar Seltzer Waters
- Canada Dry Sparkling Seltzer Water

- Lacroix Sparkling Water (a little more expensive, but still cheaper than soda).
- Waterloo (also a little more expensive, but still cheaper than soda).
- Supermarket/generic brands *sometimes* have only carbonated water and natural flavors.

100% Juices
$4.00 for ½ gallon

Okay, it's a little more expensive than a two-liter bottle of soda, but hear me out. 100% juices have vitamins C and D and minerals like potassium. Since they are high in natural sugars and, therefore, calories, the USDA recommends a limit of 1 cup (8 ounces) of 100% juice per day for adults and no more than ½ cup a day for children. Again, you can save money by sticking to these recommendations.

> Don't be fooled by juices with added sugar. Stick with 100% juices. Cranberry juice is sweetened with other juices instead of sugar now.

You can also save money by adding water to the juice so it is not so sweet. Start with 80% juice and 20% water until you are used to the taste (the family likely won't even notice the difference). Then decrease to 70% juice and 30% water until you reach a comfortable level. You can even go below 50% juice if you just want something to flavor your water. It will have the effect of adding slices of fruit, which leads to my next recommendation.

Seltzer Water Plus 100% Juice
$1.00 per 16-ounce serving

I recommend that my clients/students mix seltzer water with 100% juice as a refreshing and delicious alternative to soda, and it has helped many of them to stop drinking soda.

How to Prepare (1 minute prep time)
You will need: *100% juice, seltzer water*
1. Add about 4 ounces of 100% juice to about 12 ounces of seltzer water.
2. Add ice.
3. **Optional step:** Add lemon, lime slices, fresh herbs or your favorite fruit.

Homemade Iced Tea
$0.15 per serving (~$4 for 24 bags of tea)

The sugar added to bottled/prepared iced teas has been out of control lately. It's a good thing homemade iced tea is a thing. There are many benefits to drinking homemade iced tea:
- It tastes better.
- It is more affordable.
- No plastic leaching into the drink if you use a glass pitcher (ask for a glass pitcher as a gift if you don't have one).
- It is easy to make.
- You control what ingredients go into the drink.
- It's better for the environment.

How to Prepare (10 minutes prep time, 4 hours chill time)
You will need: *Tea bags (black, green, lemon, or your favorite), hot water*
1. Boil about 6-8 cups of water.
2. Once boiling, remove water from heat and add 3-4 tea bags.
3. Allow tea to steep for about 5 minutes.
4. Remove the tea bags.
5. **Optional step:** Add your sweetener of choice and mix.
6. Place in the fridge until cold and add ice.
7. **Optional step:** Add lemon, mint, or other fruits/herbs slices.

*Unsweetened tea is best for health, but if you want to add a little sugar/honey yourself, go for it. The important thing is that you control how much sugar/what is in your drink.

Homemade Fresh Ginger Root Tea

$0.30 per serving (~$1.00 for 4 ounces of ginger)

Several of my clients use ginger tea to keep nausea at bay or if they have an upset stomach. It has also helped some of my students with arthritic pain. But the health benefits of ginger go wildly beyond that. Ginger is packed with hundreds of phytochemicals (see Chapter 17) and has been used as an herbal medicine for centuries. Scientific studies show that ginger helps reduce inflammation and the risk of heart disease, diabetes, and stroke. It also may improve cancer symptoms and digestive health.[11]

Ginger roots' refreshing and spicy taste is a pick-me-upper in the morning or throughout the day. You can find fresh ginger root in the produce section of most grocery stores. You also can find ginger tea bags in the tea section, which is also a good option.

I regularly juice with fresh ginger root, add it to my smoothies and food, and make tea. I love strong flavors, so I add way more ginger than what is mentioned below but experiment to find out what works for you.

How to Prepare (10 minutes prep time, 4 hours chill time)

You will need: *Fresh ginger root (peeled), water, 100% honey*

1. Add 6-8 cups of water to a saucepan.
2. Add 4 square inch-long pieces (or several slices) of peeled ginger root to the water. Add more for a stronger tea.
3. Bring the water to a boil.
4. While bringing to a boil, add 3-4 tablespoons of 100% honey or your sweetener of choice.*
5. Reduce heat and simmer for about 10-20 minutes.
6. Cool the mixture, put in a glass pitcher, and refrigerate until cold.
7. **Optional step:** Strain out the ginger pieces after refrigeration.
8. **Optional step:** Add ice and or lemon slices.

*As you start to read the ingredients list more (see Chapter 13), you will notice some strange things. One of them is that some bottled and jarred honey is not all honey. For example, some companies mix honey with high fructose corn syrup, but the label says "honey." Read the ingredients list and make sure that the only ingredient is honey.

Homemade Hot Chocolate
$0.75/serving

I used to buy medium hot chocolate from a popular coffee spot on cold winter days until I realized I could make my own. The homemade version made me feel better and even helped me to move my bowels with utter ease after drinking it. I rarely go to that coffee spot for hot chocolate anymore! There are several benefits to drinking homemade hot chocolate:

- ☑ It tastes better than hot chocolate mixes.
- ☑ It's just as easy to make as the hot chocolate mixes.
- ☑ It's more affordable.
- ☑ You receive more health benefits from the cacao/cocoa.
- ☑ You control what ingredients go into your drink.

Cocoa powder costs about $0.25 per serving ($4.00-$6.00 for 8 ounces and can make about 24 cups). Cacao costs about $0.40 per serving ($8.00-$10.00 for 8 ounces or 24 servings). That is less expensive than a cup from a café or the hot cocoa mixes and chocolate syrups made with artificial ingredients and loads of sugar.

I use filtered water as my base as it reminds me of coffee without all of the caffeine and makes me feel amazing throughout the day. I used almond or whole milk, but not anymore because I don't feel as good using those options as I do with water.

Why Cacao/Cocoa, and What's the Difference?

Cacao/cocoa is an underappreciated, affordable, delicious, and healthy food. It has iron, magnesium, fiber, and powerful flavonoids/

antioxidants that evidence suggests are anti-inflammatory, protect skin from UV radiation damage, improve mood, help prevent cancer and cardiovascular disease, and promote brain health.[12] In fact, "Cocoa contains more phenolic antioxidants than most foods."[13] So, it is a delicious, easy, and affordable way to get plant-based cancer-fighting nutrients you won't find in animal products.

Cocoa powder is a more processed form of cacao powder but is still nutrient-rich and delicious. It is worth it if you can pay the extra dollars for the cacao. Nonetheless, cocoa powder is still a very good option.

How to Prepare (5 minutes)

You will need: *Cacao/cocoa, your sweetener, and your milk of choice*

1. Bring one cup of water or your milk of choice in a saucepan to a boil.
2. Add 1 or 2 teaspoons of your sweetener of choice and stir (I use maple syrup).
3. Add 1 tablespoon of 100% unsweetened cacao powder and stir.
4. Turn the heat to low while stirring *constantly* until everything is dissolved and the beverage is steaming hot (about 2 minutes).
5. **Optional step:** If you want to add extra flavor and a boost of nutrition, you can add spices like cinnamon, nutmeg, cloves, vanilla, or ginger, or experiment with your own spices.

You can also add cacao powder to smoothies for a delicious chocolatey taste and all of those wonderful health benefits.

Strategy for Reducing Sugar in Your Drink

Most of my students are shocked when I teach about the sugar/calories in popular drinks. Consider that most 16 to 20-ounce bottles of soda have anywhere from 200-300 calories from sugar.

That's about 12-19 of those little packs of sugar we get at restaurants. Also consider that 200-300 calories is about the same number of calories in a small to medium fry at a fast-food restaurant. We can easily add upward of 600 calories a day just by drinking certain beverages. And don't get me started on the big gulp-sized drinks. See Table 4.2 for information on more beverages.

— TABLE 4.2 —
SUGAR AND CALORIES IN POPULAR BEVERAGES

BEVERAGE (PER 16-OUNCE SERVING)	GRAMS OF SUGAR	TEASPOONS (PACKETS) OF SUGAR	CALORIES
Soda	59	15	240
Lemonade	58	15	240
Energy Drink	56	14	224
Frappuccino	53	13	208
Sweetened Iced Tea	48	12	192
Sports Drink	32	8	126
Vitamin-Infused Water	24	6	96

*These are actual numbers taken from the most popular brands. Check the nutrition facts label to determine how much sugar is in your drink. To convert from grams to teaspoons, divide grams by 4 (see Chapter 12 for more on these conversions).

After learning this information, many students who drink multiple sugary beverages a day declare that they are going to reduce how much they drink (or stop altogether)—even teenagers. Reducing the calories we drink in a day can be a tall order, so let's take a step-by-step approach.

In the 100% juice section, I mentioned cutting your juice with water. Cutting out sugar entirely is the ideal scenario, and some people find success in that over the long term. Many of us, however, do better over the long term by readjusting our taste slowly but surely. The process below allows for that and can be applied to all kinds of drinks, including sweetened iced teas, lemonades, sodas, hot beverages like flavored coffee, hot chocolate, and more.

For hot coffee or tea, as an example, let's say you normally add 5 teaspoons of sugar:
1. Consider adding 4.5 teaspoons instead for a week or two (or however long it takes for you to get used to that level of sweetness).
2. Allow your taste buds to adjust to 4.5 teaspoons.
3. Once adjusted, reduce to 4 teaspoons for another week or two.
4. Allow your taste buds to adjust to 4 teaspoons.
5. Then, you can reduce it to 3.5 teaspoons.
6. Then 3, 2, 1 and even zero.
7. Your taste buds will eventually adapt to less sugar.

For pre-sweetened café drinks, you can ask for 3 pumps of syrup/sweetener instead of the automatic 4 or 5 shots they may put in your drink. Or ask for 2 shots instead of 3, etc. For juices and other sugary drinks, you can add water, as mentioned in the 100% juice section.

Readjusting your tastebuds is a strategy that works for many. To readjust your tastebuds, slowly decrease the amount of sugar/sweeteners in your drinks (and food).

You can save hundreds of dollars over the course of a year by drinking the above-mentioned drinks instead of sodas and other sweetened drinks. It goes without saying that you can also save by ordering water when you go to a restaurant. I used to order water whenever I ate out because I was broke, and now that I have a few more coins, I do it because it's just healthier. Whatever your reason, you can't go wrong. The good news is that most restaurants offer filtered tap water. See Chapter 9 for more on eating out on a budget.

Not only can you save big by what you drink, but you can also save big by what you eat. Let's get into it.

CHAPTER 5

SNACKS

Snacks are another one of those under-acknowledged calorie adders. We snack throughout the day, not realizing that the calories pile on easily. A bag of chips with 200 calories here and a few mini candy bars with 200 calories there and we are pushing 400 calories just on a couple of snacks. Adding these calories to the calories from drinks, we are pushing 1,000 calories before even bringing up the calories from our meals.

I am not a big proponent of calorie counting because it can be counterproductive. However, I am a proponent of being aware of what we are taking in and making choices based on that knowledge. More on this in Part 2.

For now, below are delicious, nutritious, affordable snacks that are filled with nutrients but not a lot of calories. Most of the suggestions are grab-and-go, but some have preparation instructions. Remember, when you see ingredient quantities, they are only suggestions. Estimating quantities yourself helps you become comfortable creating meals that suit your tastes.

Fruits and Vegetables

Fruits and vegetables have nutrients called phytochemicals that are like powerful, delicious, nature-made medicines (See Chapter 17.).

They are so powerful that studies consistently show that people who eat more fruits and vegetables are healthier.[14] There is no debate about it. In fact, it is so clear that you will not find one person who will refute this claim.

If we know this about fruits and vegetables, then why don't we eat them more? A lot of it has to do with how our tastes are developed. Many of our tastes have been shaped by food manufacturers who market their highly (ultra) processed foods with lots of added sugar, salt, fat, preservatives, dyes, and other chemicals to us. Eventually, we learn to appreciate their factory-made foods more than nature-made foods.

> The USDA recommends *at least* three servings of vegetables (mostly non-starchy) *AND* at least two servings of fruit daily. Key words here: AT LEAST. Work your way up to this goal.

But, like sugary beverages, we can retrain our tastes to appreciate the wonderfulness of nature's provisions. Sometimes, it starts with doing things like putting veggies on our pizza instead of other processed toppings. Or simply snacking on fresh veggies like cherry tomatoes instead of chips to help us appreciate nature's way. This chapter includes several fruit and vegetable ideas. Take things step by step and incorporate new things at your own pace, even if it's just trying one new snack a day or week.

Eat the Fruit and Vegetable Rainbow

Eating fruits and vegetables of different colors is like taking a multivitamin because each color represents a different nutrient. Getting nutrients from nature is better than getting them from the capsules and gummies we find on the market. Why? Because the nutrients work together in the way that nature intended.

Unlike supplements, the nutrients in vegetables and fruits are embedded in a sea of other nutrients (some we have yet to identify) that work as a team to build the body. There is no way to get that type of synergy from man-made supplements.

If I were to choose one fruit and one vegetable to encourage you to start with or eat regularly, it would be any kind of berry and dark green leafy vegetables. No shade to the other fruits and vegetables, as they all pack a powerful punch. Dark berries and green leafy vegetables, just pack a more powerful one.

> To get multiple micronutrients into your diet, eat different colored fruits and vegetables, or as we dietitians like to say: **EAT THE RAINBOW.**

In-Season Fruit

$1.00/serving

The health benefits of fruit are endless, and when broken down by serving, they cost less than or just as much as other sweet treats like candy bars and cookies. Here are some tips for the best fruit deals (Also see Chapter 2.):

- ☑ **Purchase In Season.** Fruit is less expensive when purchased in the season and region in which it is grown. Most fruits, including apples, pears, plums, nectarines, watermelon, and berries, cost on average $1.00 per serving in season.
- ☑ **Purchase Bagged Fruit.** Look for the bagged fruit. It's almost always cheaper. For example, bagged apples may cost $4.00-$5.00 for 6-8 apples. That works out to $0.40- $0.50 per apple.
- ☑ **Look at Flyers.** Use flyers to see what is on sale that week.

Below are specific fruits that I highlight for their delicious taste, nutritional value, convenience, and affordability.

Bananas

$0.30/serving

Let's settle this "are bananas good for you?" debate once and for all. The answer is yes. Bananas are the most convenient and nutritious fruit year-round for the most affordable price. Even the organic is about $0.30 per banana. They are filled with potassium, which is good for regulating blood pressure, and fiber, which is good for digestion

> **Prebiotics** stimulate the growth of healthy bacteria in the gut. They are found in bananas, apples, berries, onions, garlic, and whole oats.
>
> **Probiotics** are bacteria in the gut that promote health. They are found in fermented foods and yogurt.
>
> Microorganisms in the gut are collectively known as the **microbiome**. A healthy microbiome means better metabolism, digestion, immunity and an overall healthy person.

and weight management. They also are a good source of prebiotic fiber (not to be confused with probiotics), which helps to stimulate the growth of healthy bacteria in the gut.

Bananas have a higher sugar content than other fruits, so they have gotten a bad rap. However, because they are very filling, it is hard to eat too many bananas. Just another way nature looks out for us.

Individuals who have been diagnosed with diabetes should make sure that whatever they eat fits in with their carbohydrate goals. Also, because it is important to eat the rainbow, I wouldn't recommend more than one to two bananas to save room for all those other delicious and nutritious foods and colors.

Ways to Enjoy Bananas

- Grab and go.
- Make smoothies--see below.
- Add peanut butter to banana slices.
- Add slices to oatmeal (or mush it up with oatmeal and use instead of a sweetener).

Berries (raspberries, blueberries, blackberries, strawberries)

$1.00/serving fresh ($3.00-$4.00 for four servings in season), or $0.50/ serving frozen ($4.00 for eight servings year-round)

Berries are probably the most delicious and most nutritious of all the fruits on the market. Nothing comes close. They are like little powerful balls of soldiers that go into action, fighting disease in your body on your behalf. And they are delicious. Between the antioxidants, prebiotics, potassium, and vitamin C, it doesn't get any better.

Evidence suggests that people who eat berries have a decreased risk for cancer, diabetes, cardiovascular disease, and more.[15] Also, they are one of the few foods that evidence suggests can prevent cognitive decline due to aging (other foods associated with decreased risk include citrus fruits, grapes, berries, cocoa, nuts, green tea, and coffee).[16]

> **Tip:**
> The more visible a food, the more likely we are to eat them. Put fruits and veggies in a glass container. Then place them where they are visible and easy to reach in the fridge or counter for the family to grab and go.

Strawberries (or any fruit) and Whipped Cream
$1.25/serving ($5.00 for 4 servings in season)

Berries are amazing all by themselves, however, compared to a cookie, they might not give us the same dynamic. Surprisingly, adding a little whipped cream can provide that dynamic. Whipped cream is not "healthy" by our definition; however, a serving contains less sugar, fat, and calories than a cookie or brownie.

How to Prepare (2 minutes)
You will need: *berries, whipped cream*
1. Wash and dry the berries.
2. Add washed berries to a bowl.
3. Add a spoonful of whipped cream.
4. **Optional step:** Add lemon/orange zest (see Chapter 2).

Handheld Fruits *(apples, apricots, nectarines, oranges, peaches, pears, plums, tangerines, etc.)*
$1.00-$2.00/serving

There are so many to choose from. All of these fruits have:
- ☑ Fiber, including all of the great benefits of fiber mentioned earlier. It also helps regulate blood sugar.

- ☑ Potassium, which is good for blood pressure management.
- ☑ Vitamin C, which is good for healing wounds, clearer skin, preventing colds, and cancer prevention.
- ☑ Vitamin A/carotenoids, which are good for eye health and cancer prevention.
- ☑ Phytochemicals specific to each fruit, which are good for cancer prevention and overall health.

Homemade Applesauce
$1.00/serving (1 apple per serving)

Homemade applesauce is easy, delicious, and affordable. You can eat it as is, use it to sweeten things like oatmeal, as a replacement for syrup, or as a spread for toast. This is an easy snack that adults and children can make and customize. Homemade applesauce is great because:

1. You control what ingredients go into your food.
2. There are no toxins from packaging.
3. It tastes better.
4. It is affordable.

Applesauce can be affordable and healthy if you buy it at the store. Go for the applesauce with no added sugar/other ingredients and in a glass jar for optimal health benefits. As always, check the ingredients label. It should only contain 2-3 ingredients: the fruit, maybe some ascorbic acid (or vitamin C), and water.

Experimenting with Spices Tip: Take a small spoonful of the final product and put it in a small bowl. Add your spice, mix it in, and taste. Try this with multiple spices to see what best works for you. Children like to customize their food just like adults, so let them try too!

How to Prepare (5 minutes prep time, 10 minutes cook time)

You will need: *apples, water*

1. Peel and chop a few apples, discarding the core (1 apple can serve as one serving).

2. Put the apples in a pot and add enough water to cover the apples.
3. Bring the water to a boil.
4. Cook over medium heat until the apples are soft (10-15 minutes)—add more water if necessary.
5. Mash the apples until they are chunky or smooth (whichever texture you like).
6. **Optional step:** Add a sweetener and/or spices like cinnamon (Experiment with other spices like cloves and nutmeg.).

Fruit Cups in 100% Juice
$0.75/serving (4 cups for $3.00)

Stick with the fruit cups in 100% juice if you can. These are great snacks on the go. You can also make your own fruit cups.

How to Prepare (5 minutes)

You will need: *at least 2 of your favorite fruits (see combination suggestions below)*

1. Chop 2 or more of your favorite fruits.
2. Place in glass storage containers.
   a. It may be less convenient, but it costs about the same price, tastes better, and you don't have to worry about the plastics leaching into your food.
3. **Optional step:** Add a squeeze of lemon or lime juice for a tangy twist and to help the fruit last.
4. **Optional step:** Add a few tablespoons of 100% juice.
5. Place in the fridge until you are ready to eat, or take it with you.

Here are a few great homemade fruit cup combination suggestions:
- Chopped apples, watermelon, and grapes
- Chopped pears, pineapples, and peaches
- Strawberries, blueberries, and grapes
- Chopped kiwi, blueberries, and grapes
- Chopped watermelon, pomegranate seeds, and orange slices
- Whatever you have on hand

Apples and Peanut Butter

$1.25/serving

I learned about apples and peanut butter in my home economics class in elementary school over 30 years ago, and I have been eating them ever since. They are delicious, satisfying, and convenient. You get the fiber, phytonutrients, prebiotics, vitamins, and minerals from the apple, plus all of the protein, healthy fats, vitamin E (which is a potent antioxidant), zinc, and potassium from the peanut butter. This snack is good for digestion, healthy cholesterol levels, weight management, skin, cancer prevention, and more.

How to Prepare (2 minutes)

You will need: an *apple, peanut butter*
1. Slice an apple in half and remove the core. Or you can cut the apple into slices or sticks. However, you like it.
2. Spread 2 tablespoons of peanut butter on top (or dip the slices right into the peanut butter).

Choosing a Peanut Butter

Almost every peanut butter provides protein, healthy fats, iron, magnesium, and other vitamins and minerals. Some companies add ingredients like sugar and palm oil that don't take away the nutrition but add some undesirables. For optimal health, go for the one with no more than two or three simple ingredients *that you recognize* and the lowest sugar content. If the healthiest option is outside of your budget, go with what you can afford. It will still be worth the nutrition that it provides.

You will notice that peanut butter with just peanuts and salt in the ingredients (which is typically the healthiest) will separate out the oil. If you don't like that, mix the peanut butter until the solid and liquid oil is thoroughly mixed when you open it. Put the mixed solid peanut butter in the refrigerator to keep the oil from separating out again.

Homemade Frozen Fruit Smoothies
$1.75 per 12 ounce serving

I once made fresh fruit smoothies as part of a nutrition/cooking class that I taught. One of the class participants asked, "Can I have more ice for my smoothie?" I said, "Yes." After I gave him more ice, he said, "Can I have more ice?" I said, "Of course," and he took more ice. He then said, "Ice, ice, ice, I want lots of ice. You gotta put lots of ice in the smoothies." He had the class in stitches. Needless to say, he took all the ice he wanted. The other students enjoyed the smoothies with more moderate amounts of ice and with the "ice, ice, ice."

Smoothies are an easy, affordable, and delicious way to include all kinds of nutrition in our diets. They are fun to make, and children and adults alike love them. You can make them with fresh or frozen fruit. If you use fresh fruit, be sure to include *"ice, ice, ice"* in your smoothie. Some like extra ice, even with the frozen fruit. Make it your own.

> I recommend stocking the freezer with at least one bag of frozen fruit. A 16-ounce bag that can make several smoothies costs $4.00, it lasts a long time, and it comes in handy when there is nothing else to eat. Frozen strawberries, blueberries, raspberries, mangos, blackberries—go for it.

If you don't have a blender, allow me to encourage you to get one or ask somebody for one as a gift. I have had the same blender my mother bought me for Christmas for about seven years. I make sauces, soups, smoothies, dressings, and so much more with it. It is a great investment for the kitchen, especially a healthy one.

How to Prepare (5 minutes)
You will need: *strawberries, banana, water/milk, ice*
1. Place one cup of frozen strawberries (or whatever fruit you have) in a blender.
2. Add ½ of a banana.

3. **Optional step:** Add 1 cup of another type of fruit.
4. **Optional step:** Add ½ of a ripe avocado for a creamier smoothie.
5. **Optional step:** Add ½ cup of Greek yogurt for a creamier and tangy smoothie.
6. Add 1 or 2 cups of water or your milk of choice (For a sweeter smoothie, use orange juice.).
7. If you are using fresh fruit, add ice.
8. Blend.

***Note:** If your bananas are turning brown and you don't think you can eat them all before they go bad, remove them from the peel, cut them in quarters, put them in a freezer-safe container, and freeze them. Pull them out when you are ready for a fruit smoothie.

Vegetable and Fruit Combination Ideas

- Strawberry, raspberry, and banana
- Mango and peach (my favorite)
- Raspberry and orange
- Avocado and banana
- Spinach/kale and banana
- Spinach/kale, banana, pineapple
- Spinach/kale, banana, avocado
- Spinach/kale, banana, avocado, Greek yogurt
- Spinach/kale, banana, blueberries
- Spinach/kale, peach, mango
- Carrot, mango, peach
- Carrot, apple, banana

*You can also add fresh ginger or turmeric root, two of the healthiest, disease-fighting, and delicious roots on the planet. Just make sure you remove the skin first. A small piece of fresh ginger or turmeric root costs about $0.50.

Watermelon

$0.75 per serving

$5.00-$8.00 for a whole watermelon

I have yet to meet someone who does not like watermelon. If you can find a good watermelon, just go all in. They are full of fiber, vitamin C, vitamin A, and a powerful antioxidant called lycopene, making them good for digestion, vision, and cancer prevention.

There are some tips for finding a good watermelon, like making sure it has a big yellowish-orange spot, hearing a hollow sound when you thump it, and it should be heavy for its size. You can try using these tips, but to be honest, they are not 100%. Where you get your watermelon is more important for taste than anything. Some stores just don't provide good watermelon. If yours does, be grateful. If yours doesn't, find out through the grapevine where you can get a good old-fashioned sweet and juicy watermelon.

Dates

$0.75/serving

8 ounces for $5.00

If you want to satisfy your sweet tooth, eat a date. Some of my students find that dates satisfy their sweet tooth enough that they don't crave cookies, cakes, or other unhealthy sweet treats.

Dates are filled with fiber, potassium, iron, magnesium, and protein and are highly respected foods in certain cultures around the world for their health benefits. There is even evidence to suggest that dates have anti-diabetic, anti-inflammatory, and anti-tumor activity.[17]

Dates are so sweet and high in fiber that you will only be able to eat one or two, especially if you take small bites and chew them well. Allow yourself to appreciate the sweetness and natural flavor. They make a delicious breakfast treat, sweet snack, or even dessert.

In-Season Vegetables
$1.00/serving

You want to control diabetes and blood pressure? Eat more vegetables. You want to manage your weight? Eat more vegetables. You want to prevent cancer and have better vision? Eat more vegetables. You want to have more energy and a better mood? Eat more vegetables. You want to get rid of constipation? Eat more vegetables. If you can name it, eating more vegetables more than likely can help you with it.

> People often ask me, "What is one thing that I can do to improve my health the most?" My answer is always, "Drink mostly water, eat green leafy vegetables or dark berries every day." Choose one, choose them all, but they are all powerful things you can do to improve your health instantly.

Like fruit, vegetables can be less expensive when purchased in season and are more affordable than fruit in or out of season. In fact, several veggies, such as cucumbers, celery, baby carrots, kale, broccoli, and collard greens, cost pennies on the dollar per serving any time of year.

Snacking Vegetables
$0.50-$1.00 per serving
$1.00-$1.50 per serving with dip

The best way to consume vegetables for optimal nutrition is raw. Cooked and frozen are also nutritious, but raw is best. The below snacking vegetables are great for children and adults alike.

- Baby carrots
- Baby bell peppers
- Broccoli
- Cauliflower
- Celery sticks
- Cherry/grape tomatoes
- Cucumber slices

- Bell pepper slices (the best)
- Sugar snap peas
- Zucchini slices

Feel free to dip raw vegetables in your favorite dressing (even if it is not the healthiest dip). When I am in a dipping mood, I use hummus or whatever dressing I have in the fridge. The goal is to eat vegetables and get those nutrients. The more vegetables and other healthy foods you put in your system, the less room you have for the not-so-healthy foods.

Celery and Peanut Butter
$0.75/serving
$7.00 for one celery stalk/bunch and a jar of peanut butter (about 10 servings).

This is a delicious, nutritious, convenient, and satisfying way to take the hunger edge off.

How to Prepare (2 minutes)
You will need: *celery, peanut butter*
1. Cut 2 sticks/ribs of celery in half.
2. Spread 2 tablespoons of peanut butter on the celery stick (or dip the celery right into the peanut butter).

Avocados and Crackers or Rice Cakes
$1.75/serving

Avocados have remained affordable despite the high rise in prices. At $1.50 for one (or the price of a candy bar) or a bag of 4 for $5.00, that price is hard to beat. Studies show that avocados can reduce cholesterol levels (from the healthy fats and phytosterols), improve vision (from the carotenoids), help regulate blood sugar, and are a good source of prebiotics, which can help stimulate the growth of healthy bacteria (probiotics) in the gut.[18] A healthy gut means an overall healthier person.

How to Prepare (3-5 minutes)
You will need: *avocado, crackers, salt*
1. Put your knife at the top of one avocado and poke it until you hit the hard pit in the middle.
2. Circle the knife around the avocado while touching the pit.
3. Once all the way around, twist the avocado until the two halves come apart.
4. Once open, make multiple slices along the length of ½ the avocado (leave the pit in the other half until you are ready to eat).
5. Cut the slices out of the avocado with a knife.
6. Add the avocado slices to your crackers/rice cakes.
7. Add a pinch of salt on top of the avocado.
8. **Optional step:** Slice some jalapeño peppers very thin and put them on top of the avocado.

Other Ways to Enjoy Avocados

- Slice/chop avocados, sprinkle on a little salt and enjoy.
- Add to eggs, tacos, burritos, and salads.
- Add to your favorite sandwich.
- Add to a smoothie for a nice creamy texture.
- Add them to toast with a sprinkle of salt. Add sliced tomatoes, red onions, and jalapeños for a spicy and delicious pop.
- Add to vegetable pasta dishes.
- Make guacamole…

Easy Homemade Guacamole
$1.75/serving

How to Prepare (3-5 minutes)
You will need: *avocados, salt*
1. Slice two avocados in half (see previous section).
2. Remove the pit.

3. In a small glass bowl, pinch each half of the avocado until all the flesh comes out.
4. Smash the avocados with a fork and add salt.
5. **Optional ingredients:** Add fresh finely chopped garlic (or garlic powder), finely chopped onions (or onion powder), chopped cilantro, tomatoes, jalapeños, and/or lemon or lime juice.
6. Mix.
7. Eat immediately or chill in the refrigerator for a few hours.

*If you won't be eating the guacamole right away, squeeze a little lemon juice on it and refrigerate. The vitamin C from the lemon juice helps to preserve the avocado and keep it from browning. It also tastes delicious.

Ways to Use Guacamole

- Use as a veggie dip.
- Add to crackers, rice cakes, or toast.
- Top tacos/burritos.
- Add to sandwiches.
- Top beans and rice.
- Experiment by adding it to your favorite entrée (I love adding it to baked sweet potatoes and black beans.).

You may have heard about the controversy around avocados and the human rights abuses associated with sourcing them. Unfortunately, our food industry is rife with these types of controversies. The best thing you can do is try to buy local food whenever you can, purchase food from a company with fair trade practices, and/or grow your own food to disincentivize these controversial practices. However, when these are not options, use your own moral compass to determine if you want to include them in your diet. With no guilt. Because the healthier you are, the more you have the energy and motivation to support causes that matter most to you and the type of world you want to live in.

Popcorn

$0.50/serving

I am not talking about the double cheese, butter, triple caramel dipped, with chocolate drizzle type of popcorn. I am talking plain and simple popcorn with salt, seasoning, and a little oil or even a little bit of butter. Popcorn is a great crunchy snack and alternative to things like potato chips, and cheese snacks. You can find some great-tasting quality popcorn for $2.00-$3.00 a bag still. My personal favorite is plain Skinny Pop Popcorn. They have small bags at the dollar store.

To find a healthy popcorn, look at the nutrition facts label and check for sodium, fat, and sugar. Then look at the ingredients label—make sure it has simple ingredients that you recognize. Again, see Chapter 13.

If you want to save more and be even healthier, purchase the plain kernels and pop them yourself according to the instructions on the bag. After popping the kernels, put them in a paper bag and mix them with one tablespoon of oil/butter and spices as listed below (The oil helps to make the spices stick and give the popcorn more texture and flavor.). Here are some spice combinations you might like:

- 1 tablespoon of olive oil and a pinch of salt
- 1 tablespoon of olive oil and a pinch of pepper
- 1 tablespoon of coconut oil with a pinch of cinnamon
- 1 tablespoon of coconut oil with a pinch of ground ginger and a sprinkle of sugar
- 1 tablespoon of parmesan cheese (It's not healthy but it has a lot fewer calories than other hard cheeses.).
- ½ tablespoon of butter (See more on saturated fat in chapter 15.).

- Other great spices to add include cayenne pepper, chili powder, garlic powder, smoked paprika, or your favorite spice.

Peanuts
$0.30/serving (one 16-ounce jar costs $3.00)

You can buy portioned-to-go packs of peanuts for $1.00 at corner and dollar stores. Between the protein, fiber, healthy fat, and iron, you're getting a big bang for your buck. Peanuts are high in calories, so if you are watching your calories, you will want to stick with the serving size of one ounce (which is about what you could fit into a shotglass). You can also make a trail mix with peanuts.

Sunflower or Pumpkin Seeds
$0.30/serving (16-ounce packages cost about $5.00)

When I was in high school, my classmates carried around bags of sunflower seeds and chomped on them throughout the school day. I had no idea how good they were for us until I got older.

Sunflower and pumpkin seeds are great snacks because they are filling (the protein and fiber make us less likely to desire other snacks) while providing a ton of other nutrients like B vitamins, healthy fats, vitamin E, and other cancer-fighting antioxidants. They are also sold in convenient, individual to-go packages at corner and dollar stores.

Homemade Trail Mix
$1.00/serving

Trail mixes are a delicious conglomerate of all kinds of nutrients. You get the health benefits from nuts (fiber, protein, healthy fat, cancer-fighting antioxidants) and the health benefits from dried fruit (fiber and a whole bunch of vitamins and minerals, depending on the type of fruit). One of my favorite trail mixes is nuts, raisins, and…that's it. But there are a variety of trail mixes that you can make to suit your tastes.

How to Prepare (2 minutes)
You will need: *nuts, dried fruit, seeds*
- Mix as many of the following ingredients together as you want.
  - Nuts (peanuts, cashews, pecans, pistachios, etc.)
  - Dried fruit (raisins, dried cranberries, apricots, blueberries, etc.)
  - Seeds (pumpkin, sunflower seeds, etc.)

Some people add candy and cereal, which is always an option, but nuts, dried fruits (without added sugar), and seeds are the perfect combination.

There are also lots of healthy, delicious, and affordable (especially if sticking to the serving size) trail mixes you can buy. If the price of the trail mix is a little too high, save money by making your own.

Greek Yogurt
$1.00/serving

On top of being a great source of calcium and protein, yogurt is a great source of probiotics. Recall that probiotics are microorganisms (like bacteria) that help to create a healthy gut. A healthy gut is one of the main determinants of an overall healthy person.

As always, I recommend the organic brands if they fit your budget. Non-organic Greek yogurt provides many of the same nutrients as organic; it just may come with unwanted baggage (hormones for example).

Purchase plain yogurt and add your own sweeteners/fruit/toppings (including homemade applesauce or

> **Creating personal standards for specific foods will help remove some of the stress of choosing the best option. For example, if my standard is no more than 250 grams of sodium per serving for any packaged food, I will know right away if I am going to put it back on the shelf or investigate further.**

fruit sauce). But if you don't want to worry about adding things to your yogurt and just want to grab and go, create standards for what type of yogurt you will purchase. My personal standard is that it has to have less than 15 grams of *total* sugar and should only have a few simple ingredients.

Cottage Cheese and Fruit
$1.00/serving

I often provide healthy snacks at certain of my classes for the students to try. One person in this particular class said that he hated cottage cheese when I brought it out. When he tried it with pineapple chunks, he was shocked that he liked it so much. He left the class saying that he was going to eat cottage cheese with pineapple as a snack now. He made sure to say that it would "only be with pineapples because I don't like it plain." You never know what you like unless you try different things. I found that cottage cheese and blackberries are amazing too.

Cottage cheese is a very satisfying, high-protein, high-calcium, and low-calorie snack. Cottage cheese with fruit makes a good breakfast too. Cottage cheese can be high in sodium and, like yogurt, can be high in sugar. Consider looking for the low-sodium plain versions with no added sugar and adding your own fruit.

Seaweed Snack Sheets
$1.00/serving

Seaweed is packed with fiber, potassium, iron, iodine, and phytochemicals and even has a little B12 (one of the only vitamins that you won't find in plant-based foods). You can find the little snack sheets for $1.00 a pack. They are salty, crunchy snacks that provide a lot of nutrition and taste but not a lot of calories (~25 calories per pack) and are a good alternative to chips.

Homemade Potato Chips and Salsa
$1.00/serving

Homemade potato chips can serve as an alternative to tortilla or potato chips. Here is a homemade potato chip and salsa idea that children and adults alike will love:

How to Prepare Homemade Potato Chips (5 minutes prep time, 15 minutes cook time)
You will need: *yellow or red potatoes, oil, salt*
1. Preheat oven to 375°F.
2. Slice one potato into very thin slices (leave the skin on for more fiber).
3. Coat slices with oil (about 1 teaspoon).
4. Add a sprinkle of salt.
5. Spread out slices on a baking sheet so that they do not touch.
6. Bake for 5-10 minutes in the oven (watch closely because they burn easily).
7. Remove, flip, and bake for another 5-10 minutes.
8. Turn oven to broil and cook for 1-2 minutes more so that the chips will get crunchy.

How to Prepare Homemade Salsa (5 minutes)
You will need: *tomatoes, onions, garlic, jalapeños, salt*
1. Finely chop some tomatoes, onions, garlic and jalapeños.
    a. I purposely left out quantities here. But if you want some guidance, start with one large tomato and ¼ of a small red onion, 2 cloves of garlic, and ¼ of a small jalapeño.
2. Add a pinch of salt and taste. Add more until you reach the taste you like. Garlic powder, onion powder, cumin, and chili powder are also nice spices to add using the same method.
3. **Optional step:** Add a little bit of honey. Start with 1 teaspoon and add to taste.

4. **Optional step:** Add fresh chopped cilantro and lime juice if you have some.
5. Mix, taste, and adjust ingredients accordingly.

Corn On The Cob
$0.40 per serving

Corn is a healthy, delicious, fiber-packed, affordable snack and is so easy to make. You don't need anything to cook it, no oil, no butter, no spices, no nothin'—just corn!

How to Prepare (1 minute prep time, 25-30 minutes cook time)
You will need: *ears of corn*
1. Preheat oven to 375°F.
2. Place corn on the cob on a baking sheet.
3. Bake for 15 minutes.
4. Turn the corn over and bake for another 15 minutes or until soft throughout.
5. Remove corn from the oven and enjoy.
6. **Optional step:** Add salt, pepper, cayenne pepper, or other spices.

Since I presented you with meals that contain potatoes and corn, allow me to say this about them, and let me tag on iceberg lettuce: Potatoes, corn, and iceberg lettuce are very good for us. Let me say it a little louder for the people in the back.

Potatoes, corn, and iceberg lettuce are very affordable, nutrient-rich foods. They are healthy!

If I had a dollar for the number of times people said, "Iceberg lettuce is bad for you," or "There is no nutrition in corn or potatoes," I would be rich. Thankfully though, these statements are not true—like, at all. Potatoes are filled with fiber, potassium, and B vitamins. Corn has fiber, vitamin A, potassium, magnesium, iron, and a bunch of B vitamins. Iceberg lettuce has fiber, vitamin K, vitamin C, vitamin A, and a bunch of B vitamins. They also have powerful phytochemicals.

Potatoes get a bad rap because we eat them in the form of French fries and potato chips. Corn gets a bad rap because people think it's just carbohydrates and nothing else. Iceberg lettuce gets a bad rap because it's not as nutrient-rich as kale or collard greens. While two out of three of these are true (the corn story is false), none of it means the food is unhealthy. How you eat them and how much you eat makes all the difference.

Yes, you can choose iceberg lettuce and feel good about it. Yes, you can eat roasted potatoes and feel good about it. Yes, you can eat corn on the cob and feel that you are doing something great for your body. The bonus is that corn costs $0.40 an ear; potatoes, about $1.00 a large potato; and iceberg lettuce, about $2.00 for a whole bunch of salad servings. Don't miss out.

Homemade Plantain Chips
$0.30/serving

Plantains are like large bananas, only they have more starch, calories, and fiber per serving, do not spike blood sugar as much, and are usually cooked. They make a good hardy snack, side dish, or even dessert if you prepare them with coconut oil.

The riper the plantain the sweeter the taste. The greener the plantain, the more prebiotics you will have to promote the healthy bacteria in the gut. Whether very ripe (yellow) or less ripe (green), you will get potassium, vitamin A, B vitamins, magnesium, and more. Nutrients that are good for the heart, eyes, brain, and immune system.

All you need is ripe plantains (one plantain makes 2 servings), just enough oil to coat the plantains, and your favorite seasonings. No seasoning is necessary; however, salt, garlic powder, and chili powder work well for savory plantains. Cinnamon works well with coconut oil for sweet plantains (no sugar necessary, trust). And like always, you can experiment with your favorite spices.

How to Prepare (5 minutes prep time, 20 minutes cook time)
You will need: *ripe plantains, your oil of choice, salt*
1. Preheat oven to 400°F.
2. Cut 1 large plantain into ¼-inch slices (for two servings).
3. Coat plantain slices lightly with your favorite oil (about 1 teaspoon).
4. **Optional step:** Add a sprinkle of your favorite spices.
5. Place coated slices on a baking sheet, making sure they do not touch (Use parchment paper if you have it.).
6. Put in the oven for 10 minutes.
7. Flip and bake for another 5-10 minutes until plantains have a brown coating on both sides and are cooked throughout.

Sweet plantains with a meal can help curb the sugar cravings typical after eating a savory meal. Alternatively, you can even eat them for dessert.

There are also several easy, healthy, plantain recipes online. This one happens to be my favorite for its ease, health benefits, and taste.

Homemade 100% Fruit Juice Popsicles
$0.50/serving

Put popsicles or freezies (some call them icies) made with 100% fruit juice in the freezer. They are delicious, can curb a sweet tooth, don't have a lot of sugar or calories, and even bring some vitamin C free-radical boosting action (which helps to prevent cancer). There are several healthy popsicles on the market made with real fruit and no added sugar. It is also easy and more affordable to make your own. All you need is your favorite 100% juice and a popsicle mold. The stainless-steel molds are the best for health but go with what suits your wallet.

How to Prepare (1 minute prep time, overnight in freezer)
You will need: *100% juice, popsicle mold*
1. Pour 100% juice (my favorite is grape juice) into the popsicle mold.
2. Place in the freezer overnight.

Healthy snacking can make a difference in the diet, even if you don't change anything else. Chapter 11 has more information on setting small goals that lead to bigger goals. One small goal could be to replace one unhealthy snack per day with a healthy snack. It may not seem like much, but, as you know, small changes make a big difference. For example, swapping out that piece of cake for dessert with sweet homemade plantain chips can save calories and provide health-boosting nutrition that you would not get from the cake. It makes a difference.

The snacks in this chapter are the tip of the iceberg when it comes to healthy, affordable snacks. Doing an internet search for healthy, affordable snacks will turn up several easy and delicious recipes. You can also borrow books from the library for more ideas. Everything labeled healthy is not always healthy, so use Part 2 to help you determine if it is, in fact, healthy. Do the same for breakfast, lunch, and dinner ideas. Let us continue with breakfast.

CHAPTER 6

BREAKFAST

When I was in graduate school, I had a professor who would always tout the benefits of eating breakfast, especially when it came to weight management. There are claims that breakfast helps regulate blood sugar levels better throughout the day, boost metabolism, increase productivity, and improve concentration levels. Some scientific literature suggests that these claims are true, other literature suggests that they are not. What is undeniably true about breakfast is that:

- ☑ It provides us with energy, which is important for moving, thinking and productivity.
- ☑ What we eat for breakfast has a lot to do with whether/how we benefit from breakfast.

Everyone is different and what works for one person may not work well for another person. This is why it is important for us to listen to our bodies when our bodies speak to us.

Some of my students tell me that eating a piece of fruit and yogurt works well for them. Others like to make their own juice or smoothies in the morning. I love the feeling I get after eating grapefruit or berries in the morning. It awakens my senses, fills me up and gives me that *I can take on the world* type energy. I then like to eat a fiber and protein-rich snack, like nuts, mid-morning, which sets me up well for a nice lunch.

Despite their popularity, highly processed foods like bagels, donuts, pancakes, and even granola bars will likely make us feel sluggish shortly after eating them and will raise blood sugar levels more than foods with fiber and protein.

> You can eat whatever you want for breakfast. It does not have to be traditional breakfast foods.

I recommend eating a fiber and/or protein-rich breakfast every morning to fill you up with nutrients and get you going. This chapter presents some recommendations that fit this bill. While some of these breakfast options are traditional, some are not. Breakfast is only defined by the approximate time period in which it is eaten, not the actual food itself. Breakfast food does not have to be eggs and oatmeal, although those are good too!

Allow me to remind you to look up a food pantry or food distribution in your area. You will find several of the food items mentioned below at many of these distributions.

Creamy Oatmeal Your Way
$0.30/serving

Oatmeal consumption is associated with lower cholesterol levels, healthy weight management, and blood sugar control. I cook oatmeal with water, sweeten it with either honey or fruit, and add cinnamon (gotta have cinnamon) and pecans or walnuts. But you can dress it up with all kinds of things: fruit, nuts, raisins, dried cranberries, nut butter, applesauce, or whatever your heart desires. A surprisingly good oatmeal is plain oatmeal, water, and smushed bananas.

How to Prepare (5 minutes prep time, 5-10 minutes cook time)

You will need: *oatmeal, water, your sweetener of choice, your topping of choice*

1. Add oatmeal to water in a saucepan (1 cup water for every ½ cup of oatmeal typically works well).

2. Add your sweetener of choice.
3. **Optional steps:** Add a pinch of salt, fresh/frozen fruit, nuts, cinnamon, or other spices.
4. Stir and allow the oatmeal and ingredients to meld together into a porridge-like consistency. Add more water for thinner oatmeal.

*You can also use milk instead of water or steel-cut oats instead of rolled oats. Steel-cut oats are less processed but cost a bit more and require more time to cook. They are better nutritionally, especially for individuals who may have diabetes or are trying to watch their weight. Still, eating rolled oats (even the instant ones) has plenty of benefits. And as always, I recommend organic if your budget permits.

Oat Bites
$0.50/serving

These are a good substitute for donuts and danishes in the morning. You get all of the health benefits from the oats, they are very easy to make, and you can eat them on the go. This is a snack that children love to make and eat also.

How to Prepare (5 minutes prep time, 1-2 hours in the fridge)
You will need: *oatmeal, peanut butter, honey, salt*
1. Mix oatmeal, peanut butter, a little bit of honey, and a pinch of salt in a bowl until thoroughly mixed (1 cup of oatmeal to ½ cup of peanut butter works but remember to taste and adjust to suit your palate).
2. **Optional step:** Add seeds, nuts, spices, chocolate chips, and/or shredded coconut and fold in.
3. Put the mixture in the fridge for at least an hour.
4. Scoop out balls of the mixture and roll them into a ball.
5. Eat right away or put back in the fridge to enjoy another time.

Baked Sweet Potato
$1.00/serving

This is a surprisingly delicious and filling breakfast, especially in the fall and winter months. It is also great for lunch or dinner. Sweet potatoes are one of the most delicious, affordable, nutrient-rich foods on the planet. They are filled with fiber to fill you up, vitamin A for good vision, vitamin E for glowing skin, vitamin C to prevent colds and fight cancer, potassium for blood pressure control, antioxidants, again, to prevent cancer, and are a steady source of energy throughout the morning. Even though they are sweet, they don't spike your blood sugar because of the fiber. Also, because they are sweet, they take care of that sweet craving making us less likely to reach for the sweet treats.

They are not the highest source of protein, so if you want to heat up some black beans sprinkled with salt and add, it is a surprisingly delicious combination. There is a lot of fiber between the black beans and sweet potatoes, it will help to clean you out. Embrace it. Pooping regularly is a very good thing.

How to Prepare (5 minutes prep time, 35-45 minutes cook time)
You will need: *sweet potato, oil, salt*
1. Preheat oven to 400°F.
2. Wash and scrub a sweet potato(es).
3. Poke the sweet potatoes with a fork making multiple holes.
4. Coat potatoes in your oil of choice (about 1 teaspoon).
5. Place on a baking sheet and bake for about 35-45 minutes.

Prepare first thing in the morning and by the time you are dressed, your breakfast will be ready. You can also prepare the day before and heat it up in the morning. Eat the yummy skin too. It adds more fiber. Remember, you can add toppings, like black beans or guacamole (my favorite combination that I often eat for dinner with some sauteed onions and peppers). Or you can add a little cinnamon and your sweetener of choice. But they are good without any additions.

Leftover Beans and Brown Rice or Quinoa
$1.00/serving

I lived in Costa Rica with a host family one winter, and I was amazed at how healthy the people there cooked. It was always fresh fruits, vegetables, and always beans. In fact, their national dish is called Gallo Pinto and is basically rice beans, onions, and other vegetables and spices. It was so popular that we would eat Gallo Pinto for breakfast.

At the time I was there, the Costa Rican government did a lot of work to preserve their natural lands, and it seemed like the people I was around ate natural foods more than processed foods, even though processed foods were available.[19] Beans can set you up for a great morning, making you less likely to go for processed foods. Be sure to use brown rice (white rice can cause one to crash mid-morning). Or try quinoa in place of rice. Chapter 8 has more information on using quinoa.

Baked Home Fries
$0.75/serving

I will reiterate that potatoes have several important nutrients and are very healthy, especially if you eat the skin and bake them instead of fry them. Eat these home fries any time of the day as they also make a great side dish for dinner. Add some roasted onions and peppers and you have yourself a delicious nutrient-rich breakfast. You can add an egg (scrambled or hard boiled) for protein. Potatoes have a lot of carbohydrates, so as with all things starchy, watch portion sizes.

How to Prepare (5 minutes prep time, 20-30 minutes cook time)

You will need: *potatoes, oil, salt, your favorite spices*
1. Preheat oven to 400°F.

2. Wash/scrub potato(es) (Use one small potato for one serving.).
3. **Optional step:** Peel the potatoes (leave the skin on for more fiber).
4. Cut up potatoes into evenly sized cubes.
5. **Optional step:** For crispier fries, throw the cubed potatoes into boiling water for 5 minutes, drain and dry the potatoes well.
6. Lightly coat potatoes with your oil of choice (about ½ teaspoon per potato).
7. Add pepper, salt, or other spices/herbs. Rosemary, thyme, cayenne pepper, and garlic powder are some of my favorites.
8. Spread out potatoes on a baking sheet and bake for 10 minutes.
9. Flip cubes at 10 minutes with a spatula and cook for another 10 minutes or until golden brown and cooked throughout.

*If you want to add roasted onions and bell peppers to this meal, you can roast the potatoes, onions, and pepper on the same baking dish.

Egg Muffins with Veggies
$1.00/serving

Eggs were another popular breakfast item in Costa Rica. There are pros and cons to eating eggs. While I believe that the pros outweigh the cons, I suggest limiting egg consumption to no more than one to two eggs a day (See Chapter 15 for more on eggs.).

These homemade egg muffins are delicious and easy to make. They are packed with protein, vitamin D, vitamin A, and choline. Choline is very important for brain health and vitamin D is believed to prevent a multitude of diseases, including cancer, and is important for bone health. You also get fiber, vitamins, and minerals from the vegetables you include in your muffins. You can prepare these muffins the day before or in the morning. Children can help make these and they love to eat them also.

How to prepare (5-10 minutes of prep time, 10-15 minutes to bake)

You will need: *eggs, whatever veggies you have in the fridge, oil, salt, pepper, a muffin tin*

1. Preheat oven to 375°F.
2. Crack eggs in a bowl and whisk with a fork (one egg makes about two muffins).
3. Add finely chopped veggies (onions, peppers, spinach, jalapenos, whatever you have).
4. Add salt and pepper and mix.
5. Brush oil into a muffin tin.
6. Pour the egg mixture into the greased muffin tin (do not fill each space more than halfway).
7. Bake for 10-15 minutes until cooked throughout.

Hard Boiled Eggs, Sliced Avocado, and Tomato
$1.50/serving

When all else fails, hard-boiled eggs come to the rescue. The nutrients in avocado help to reduce inflammation and manage weight, blood pressure, cholesterol, and blood sugar levels. Add tomato slices for a refreshing and delicious dose of antioxidants that help to prevent cancer.

How to Prepare (5-10 minutes prep time, 20 minutes cook time)

You will need: eggs, salt, pepper, avocado, tomato

1. Place eggs in a pot of water and bring to a boil.
2. Once boiling, turn the heat down to a simmer and allow to cook for 10-15 minutes.
3. While the eggs are boiling, slice the avocado and tomatoes and put on a plate.
4. When the eggs are done, peel, slice, and place them over the avocado and tomatoes.
5. Sprinkle with salt and pepper.

Greek Yogurt Parfait
$1.50/serving

I listed Greek yogurt under snacks; adding a few nutrient-rich foods can turn yogurt into a hearty meal. Be careful with granola. Some brands may have over 15 grams of sugar per serving, chemicals, and artificial ingredients.

How to Prepare (3 minutes)
You will need: plain Greek yogurt, granola, your favorite fruit
1. Add ¼ cup of yogurt in the bottom of a cup or bowl.
2. **Optional step:** Before making the parfait, add a pinch of spices like cinnamon or nutmeg to the yogurt and mix well.
3. Add ¼ cup of granola cereal.
4. Add ¼ cup of yogurt on top of the granola cereal
5. Add your favorite fruit.
6. **Optional step:** Add pecans and walnuts.

Using vegan versions of yogurt is an option. Be mindful that each type brings a different nutrient profile to the table and other sets of issues. For example, plain yogurt made with coconut milk has more calories and less protein than whole milk. At the same time, it has more fiber and does not have any antibiotics or hormones like non-organic yogurts are likely to have. See Chapter 14 for the pros and cons of choosing plant-based milks.

Chia Seed Pudding
$1.25/serving

Chia seeds are seeds that become delicious and gooey when allowed to soak in milk. The seeds are filled with fiber, protein, antioxidants, vitamins, and minerals. These components are good for heart health, diabetes, cancer prevention, and weight management. The star of the chia seed is its omega-3 fat content. Omega-3s are healthy fats known for anti-inflammatory properties (which manifest as arthritis relief, for example) and their role in brain health. See chapter 17 for more information on omega-3s.

One tablespoon of chia seeds contains more than 100% of the recommended omega-3s for the day. One 12-ounce (28 tablespoons) bag costs $6.00-$8.00. Making them about $0.50 per serving.

Had I only tried this pudding as a thick pudding that you eat with a spoon, I would have written it off as a food that I do not like. However, I tried it as a loose drink instead of a thick pudding by adding more milk and it turns out that I love it that way. This is why trying different things and tailoring foods to our taste is important. We could be missing out on delicious, affordable, and healthy options!

How to prepare (5 minutes prep time, 2-8-hour fridge time)

You will need: *chia seeds, water or milk, sweetener, sealed glass container*

1. Add your sweetener of choice to a glass jar (1 teaspoon for one serving). My favorite, from a pure flavor standpoint, is maple syrup. It is more expensive, but again, if you don't use it a lot, it lasts a very long time.
2. Add your water or your milk of choice and mix (Add 1 cup for a thin beverage like pudding; for a thicker pudding, add less milk.).
3. Put chia seeds in the water/milk (1 tablespoon makes one serving).
4. Seal the jar/container and shake until the ingredients are thoroughly mixed.
5. Put in the fridge for at least 2 hours.
6. **Optional step:** When ready to eat, add berries and nuts.

*Make the pudding the night before to enjoy in the morning. You can also mix cacao powder with the sweetener for a chocolatey pudding. Or just add water and lemon or lime juice and enjoy.

Homemade Smoothies

$2.00/serving

Smoothies are a good snack and breakfast option. If you don't have a blender, ask a family member or friend to get you one as a gift.

Add vegetables like spinach, kale, and carrots to your smoothie. See Chapter 5 for smoothie instructions and fruit/veggie combination recommendations.

* * *

Anything listed in the snack, lunch, and dinner sections is fair game for breakfast. As I mentioned in the snack section, these options are something to get you started. Find other healthy, affordable, and delicious ideas online or at the library, and use the information in this book to determine whether it is healthy.

What you eat in the morning can significantly impact how you feel and what you eat throughout the day. If you are not used to eating breakfast, start with a piece of fruit or a vegetable. Sometimes, if I am on the go, I eat a bunch of cherry tomatoes or cucumber slices, which is very satisfying and refreshing. Then, I will eat a protein-rich snack, like nuts, later in the morning.

Allow your breakfast to set you up for high energy levels, a productive morning and a healthy lunch-which is what we are going to talk about next.

CHAPTER 7

LUNCH

A good breakfast will set you up for a good lunch. If you haven't eaten a good breakfast, you are likely to be ravenous by the time you get to lunch. Which also means that you will more than likely want to eat more. And the only thing that will seem to fit the bill will be heavy, fatty foods that my family and friends call "real food." Because, of course, according to some of them, fruits, veggies, and salads are not real foods.

On the other hand, if you eat a good breakfast and a healthy mid-morning snack and drink water, you won't be as hungry at lunchtime. In that case, fruits, veggies, beans, nuts, and seeds might be exactly what you need to satisfy you and give you the energy you need for the rest of the day. Pay attention to what works for you when trying different things because everybody is different.

Berries or grapefruit are the best breakfast for me in the morning because they give me all kinds of energy and feel-goods. By mid-morning, I usually want a protein-rich snack. By lunchtime, if I am not too busy, I will have something like a salad or bean tacos for lunch. If I am too busy, I will eat veggies and hummus or dried mango or something like that. Notice that I don't always eat full meals for breakfast and lunch because I like to graze for most of the day. Then I will eat a full dinner meal, which works well for me.

Instead of a full lunch, it might be better for you to snack every couple of hours. Perhaps you like eating full meals with no snacks in between or lighter meals with snacks in between. Whatever you do, try to avoid being ravenous at any point throughout the day.

A Few Things to Note About the Lunch and Dinner Ideas That Follow

- ☑ You will notice that I provide alternatives to bread and pasta. That is because bread and pasta are highly processed foods that often add calories and not many nutrients other than carbohydrates. Whole grain bread and pasta contain fiber, healthy fats, and B vitamins, which are not found in refined/white grains, so I highly recommend 100% whole grains. However, even whole grains often have an overload of carbohydrates and calories and should be eaten in moderation.
- ☑ I am also heavy-handed on the vegetarian (sometimes vegan) options. I am not trying to convert you to become a vegetarian or vegan. In fact, I eat chicken once in a while and when I travel home to Buffalo, New York, I eat the best pizza in the world with pepperoni, gluten-laden dough, cheese, and all. So, I am not a strict vegetarian, but 95% of the snacks/meals that I eat are vegetarian. And I choose this way for health, environment, and animal cruelty reasons. And yes, a part of me wants to promote that, but more importantly, my goal is to provide you with the most nutrient-rich AND affordable options—which are more likely than not to be vegetarian.

Fresh Salad Your Way

$2.00/serving

Many of my students/clients find that adding a fresh/dried fruit or a sweet dressing to salad helps curb their cravings for sweets. They also acknowledge salad as an easy and affordable way to incorporate vegetables into their food routine. A bag of spinach costs $4.00 on the high end and provides 4 salad servings. A head of lettuce runs about $3.00 a head and provides about eight servings. A bunch of kale/collard greens runs about $2.00 a bunch and provides about eight servings.

How to Prepare (10 minutes prep time)

You will need: *greens, whatever vegetables or fruit that you have in the fridge, a protein source (like beans or nuts), your favorite salad dressing (I won't be picky here.).*

1. Choose your greens (e.g., spinach, arugula, kale, lettuce [*including iceberg*], cabbage, etc.).
    a. If you use kale, wash well and massage the leaves with a little bit of oil and lemon juice. Then slice the leaves thin.
2. Add your favorite chopped vegetables (e.g. carrots, cucumbers, tomatoes, onions, peppers, beets, radishes, zucchini, etc.).
3. Add your protein (beans, nuts, seeds, hard-boiled eggs, tuna, grilled chicken, etc.).
4. Add your favorite fruit (e.g., berries, apples, pears, grapes, raisins, dried cranberries, etc.).
5. Add your favorite dressing (you can make your own–see below).
6. **Optional step:** If you grow herbs yourself, chop some parsley or cilantro into tiny pieces and mix into your salad. It adds a nice flavor burst.
7. **Optional step:** Add spices like pepper and onion powder for more flavor.

Nutrition Notes:

- A fatty salad dressing allows for better absorption of the fat-soluble vitamins A, K, E and D. See below for an easy, delicious, healthy, and affordable salad dressing.
- Squeezing lemon/citrus juice on your spinach allows for better iron absorption.

Easy Homemade Vinaigrette

$0.25 per serving

I prepared this salad dressing with high school students, and they were shocked at how easy it was to make and how delicious it was.

How to Prepare (5 minutes, prep time)

You will need: *olive oil, balsamic or apple cider vinegar, honey*

1. Mix olive oil, vinegar, and honey in a jar and shake.
    a. Start with one part oil to vinegar. That is if you add ¼ cup olive oil add ¼ cup vinegar. Then add a little bit of honey.
2. Adjust the ingredients to your liking.
    a. I like my dressing with more olive oil and less vinegar, and I prefer extra virgin olive oil and balsamic vinegar, but any oil or vinegar will work.
3. **Optional step:** Add lemon juice or black pepper.

Salad Combination Recommendations

- ☑ Kale (don't forget to rub it with oil and slice it thin), large apple chunks, raisins/dried cranberries (or fresh grapes), walnuts, and the easy homemade vinaigrette mentioned.
- ☑ Arugula, beets, thinly sliced red onions, walnuts, feta cheese, and the easy homemade vinaigrette mentioned earlier.
- ☑ Mixed greens, chopped bell peppers, carrots, cucumbers, sesame seeds, black beans, dried cranberries/raisins, finely chopped fresh parsley, your favorite dressing.

*Purchase organic produce if you can. See Chapter 2 for produce with the least and most pesticides. If organic is outside your budget right now, focus on the Clean Fifteen.

Easy Tacos
$1.00/taco

Everybody loves tacos, and with a well-stocked pantry, the only thing you will need to purchase for these tacos are fresh vegetables. Children can help with making these. They also love to eat them.

How to Prepare (20 minutes prep time, 45-60 minutes cook time for beans)

You will need: *taco shells/tortillas, rice,* b*lack/pinto beans, onion,* bell peppers, tomatoes, s*alsa, your favorite lettuce/leafy green,* salt, pepper, cumin, onion powder, garlic powder, cayenne pepper (**Optional:** *Avocado slices, bell peppers slices, corn, sour cream, shredded cheese, fresh cilantro*)

1. Cook the rice (Cook ½ cup for 1-2 people or 1.5 cups for a family of four).
   a. Rinse and cook rice according to package instructions.
2. Cook the beans (1 cup for 1-2 people or 2 cups for a family of four).
   a. Rinse and cook beans according to package instructions.
   b. Drain the beans when they are ready but save the starchy bean water (or save the starchy water from the rice).
   c. Add about ½ cups of starchy water to the beans and mash some of them, leaving some of them whole.
   d. Add the spices (start with ½ teaspoons of salt, ¼ teaspoons of pepper, 1 teaspoon of cumin), and mix. Taste and add more seasonings to your taste. You can also use your favorite taco seasoning brand.
   e. Allow the mashed/whole beans mix to cook on low for 5 minutes. Add more of the starchy water for more soupy beans.

3. While the beans and rice are cooking, cut 1 onion and 1 green bell pepper into thin slices and sauté. You can also use raw onions and peppers. *Increase or decrease the quantity of peppers and onions based on how many you are cooking for.*
4. Chop any other vegetables you'd like to use including tomatoes, avocado, jalapeños, lettuce, etc.
5. Start building your taco:
    a. Add the rice and beans to the taco shell. You can also make a taco bowl without a shell or tortilla.
    b. Add the raw or sautéed onions and peppers.
    c. Add the fresh vegetables.
    d. **Optional step:** Make homemade guacamole and salsa and add.
    e. **Optional step:** Add fresh chopped cilantro (from your herb garden if you have one).
    f. **Optional step:** Add sour cream or cheese.

Notes:
- ☑ You are always welcome to add a meat-based protein source, but these are delicious as is.
- ☑ Be aware, 1 cup of dried rice or beans is actually 3 cups cooked. Cook according to need. If you wind up cooking too much, save the leftovers for another dish.

Personalized Snack Tray
$2.00/serving

If food is easily accessible, I am going to eat it. So not only do I have a fruit basket with apples, oranges, and bananas, but I also wash a few berries, put them in a glass bowl, and leave the bowl on the counter. If you don't eat them up quickly, I recommend putting them in the fridge where they are visible and easily accessible. And this is how my snack tray sometimes develops for lunch.

1. Put some berries (or whatever other fruit is available) on a plate.
2. Add a vegetable (like sliced cucumbers, cherry tomatoes, celery sticks).
3. Add some nuts (or a few small slices of cheese for protein).
4. Add a few crackers.
5. **Optional step:** Add a dip like hummus or ranch for your veggies.

Notes:
- ☑ Crackers and cheese are highly processed and fall into that "unhealthy with redeeming qualities" category mentioned in the introduction. You'll want to stick to the serving sizes on the package. Also, look for crackers that have simple ingredients. Plain Triscuits have wheat, canola oil, and salt, for example.

Tuna Fish Salad and Veggies
$1.50/serving

Okay, tuna is not a vegetarian choice, but it has many health benefits, is low in calories, goes well with veggies, is easy to make, most people love it, and is affordable. One $2.00 can of tuna fish is enough for two servings. Beware that the recommendation for fish is no more than two servings a week. Also, there are some mock tuna fish recipes that you can create using chickpeas that are surprisingly delicious. There are multiple versions online that you can search for.

How to Prepare (10 minutes prep time)
You will need: *one can of tuna, celery, onions, salt, pepper*
1. Drain tuna and put it in a glass bowl.
2. Add finely chopped celery and onion (about ¼ cup for each can of tuna).
3. Add pepper and salt.

4. **Optional step:** Add 1-2 tablespoons of your favorite mayo.
5. **Optional step:** Add fresh dill (from your garden if you have one) or dried dill.
6. **Optional step:** Add 1 tablespoon of relish.
7. Mix all ingredients and add ingredients to taste.
8. Eat with:
    a. Baby carrots
    b. Cucumber slices
    c. Cherry tomatoes
    d. Avocado slices
    e. Apple slices
    f. Jalapeño slices
    g. Rice cakes (instead of bread)
    h. Wrap in large lettuce or collard green leaves for a wrap
    i. Try an open-face sandwich by adding tuna mixture to one slice of bread instead of two

Lettuce/Collard Green Wraps

$2.00-$3.00 per serving, depending on your filling

Years ago, a student once told me she uses collard greens instead of bread for some wraps and sandwiches. Since then, I've been seeing greens and lettuce wraps in various restaurants. Even some burger places provide lettuce or greens as an option instead of bread for their burgers. Since they don't market that option much, you can always ask if that is an option.

Using lettuce and collard greens instead of bread is a swap that has tremendous health benefits (and it's easier on the wallet). Bread is highly processed and is associated with weight gain and blood sugar spikes. Collard greens and lettuce are associated with stable blood sugar and blood pressure, better vision, and brain health. There is no better swap; well, there is water for soda, and then there are berries for candy bars—ok, maybe there are equally good swaps, but you get the point.

Try lettuce or collard green leaves as wraps for one of your favorite sandwich recipes, and see what you think.

<u>How to Prepare (10 minutes prep time)</u>

You will need: *large lettuce leaves, your sandwich filling*
1. Wash collard green/lettuce leaves well (butterhead or romaine are good large lettuce leaves).
2. Add your sandwich content to the middle of the leaf. Could include:
    a. Hummus, avocado, cucumbers, feta cheese, and vinaigrette
    b. Tuna salad
    c. Grilled chicken strips, avocado, spinach, and your favorite dressing
3. Roll up the leaf.

* * *

Again, these are just a few ideas to get you started. Search for other healthy, affordable lunch ideas online or at the library.

Any breakfast food can be lunch, even outside of the brunch setting. Also, leftovers from the night before are a popular, affordable lunch option. So, let's get into some dinner ideas that you can also eat for lunch the next day.

CHAPTER 8

DINNER

Some of my students like big breakfasts, small lunches, and even smaller dinners. Others like small breakfasts, big lunches, and even bigger dinners. Some like to snack throughout the day. However, one consistency is that they prefer not to eat a few hours before bed.

Some say it helps them sleep better; others say it helps with weight management. Others say that they feel less groggy in the morning, and others say that it leaves them with a healthy appetite in the morning and that they are more likely to eat breakfast.

Leaving a 2–3 hour window between dinner and bedtime allows your body to focus on rejuvenating itself while sleeping. You don't want your body to worry about digesting food while it is rejuvenating, do you?

Of course, the type of dinner you eat also makes a difference, and taken together, these things can set you up for success the next day.

With all of these benefits, one can argue dinner is the most important meal of the day. But who's competing? Not breakfast!

> Good dinner hours before bed →
> Better sleep →
> Better mood →
> Mood/appetite for a good breakfast →
> More energy →
> More productivity →
> Less stress

These tips will help you maximize the benefits of eating dinner:
- ☑ Eat dinner at least 2-3 hours before going to bed.[20]
- ☑ Eat whole food proteins and vegetables (for fiber) that will keep you full for the evening.
- ☑ Pay attention to portion sizes.
- ☑ Chew your food well and eat slowly. This will help you feel fuller with less food and allow your digestive system to work its magic best.[21]

The following dinner suggestions have whole vegetarian proteins and vegetables to help fill you up so that you won't feel the need to eat more before bed.

After Dinner

If you want dessert after dinner, eat a piece of fruit (add a few pecans/walnuts and top with whipped cream if you want), baked plantains, a fruit smoothie, an oatmeal bite, chia seed pudding, or unsweetened dried fruit. These are all mentioned in Chapter 5.

If you are not sensitive to caffeine, try the cup of homemade hot chocolate mentioned in Chapter 4 or a piece of dark chocolate to satisfy your sweet tooth.

Black Bean Patties and Homemade French Fries
$1.00/serving

I don't buy burgers at the grocery store unless they are vegetarian. So, I had no idea how much beef patties, turkey burgers, and other meat-based burgers cost. I often complained about the cost of my favorite store-bought black bean burgers (4 for $6.00 or 8 for $8.00 depending on the brand). The other day, I strolled by the freezer section and saw "seasoned turkey burgers"—$12.99 for a six-pack. I am sorry, how much? Next to the turkey burgers were the Angus burgers—$14.99 for 6 burgers. I thought to myself, "I know it's cheaper to be a vegetarian, but these are better savings than I thought." Needless to say, I don't complain about the price of my black bean burgers anymore.

I compared the nutrition information of the turkey, Angus, and black bean burgers. The information in Table 8.1 is what I found. The turkey patties have 270 fewer calories, 13.5 fewer grams of saturated fat, 260 fewer milligrams of sodium, and 7 more grams of protein than the Angus beef patty. So, the vegetarian option costs less than both animal products, but also the healthier animal option (the turkey) costs less than, the less healthy option (the Angus beef).

— TABLE 8.1 —
COST AND NUTRIENT COMPARISON BETWEEN STORE-BOUGHT ANGUS BEEF BURGERS AND TURKEY BURGERS

PER PATTY	ANGUS BEEF PATTIES	TURKEY PATTIES	BLACK BEAN BURGERS
Cost	$2.50	$2.17	$1.00
Calories	430	160	160
Saturated fat	15 grams	1.5 grams	1 gram
Cholesterol	110 milligrams	125 milligrams	0 milligrams
Sodium	680 milligrams	420 grams	230 milligrams
Protein	24 grams	31 grams	5 grams

There are some good veggie burger options in the frozen section. These are burgers made with vegetables and beans, not meat substitutes. To save more money, try these easy-to-make black bean burgers. Children can help make them, and they love to eat them, too.

How to Prepare Black Bean Burgers (10 minutes prep time, 10 minutes cook time)
(Add 60 minutes if using dried beans)
You will need: *black beans, fresh garlic, onions, salt, pepper, an egg*
1. Preheat oven to 375°F.

2. Add the following to a bowl:
    a. 2 cups of cooked or canned black beans for about 4-6 patties
    b. Minced garlic or garlic powder (I like lots of garlic, most people use 2-3 cloves, but I use more.)
    c. 1 small onion (You can sauté, chop, or grate them— I like grating best.)
    d. Salt and pepper
    e. **Optional step:** Add a sprinkle of breadcrumbs
    f. **Optional step:** Add cumin, black pepper, cayenne pepper, garlic powder, smoked paprika, or any other of your favorite spices
    g. 1 egg
3. Mix all of the ingredients together.
4. Form 4-6 patties with the mixture.
5. Spread a little oil on a baking sheet and place the patties on it.
6. Bake for 10 minutes. Flip and bake for another 10 minutes until cooked throughout.
7. **Optional step:** Add cheese and bake for another 3 minutes.
8. **Optional step (fixings):** Add raw onion slices, tomatoes, lettuce, mustard, sauteed mushrooms, jalapeños, avocado slices, or your favorite condiment.

*Remember, you can also use a large leafy green or lettuce leaves instead of bread. And don't forget the homemade fries!

How to Prepare Homemade French Fries (5 minutes prep time, 30 minutes cook time)

You will need: *yellow or red potatoes, oil, salt*
1. Chop up a few potatoes into the shape of French fries.
2. See Chapter 1 for roasting vegetables instructions. You can also use these instuctions for sweet potato, yuca, or zucchini fries. If making yuca fries, boil the fries for 10 minutes before baking.

Split Pea Soup
$1.25/serving

Split pea soup is a delicious meal all by itself. Split peas are filled with protein, healthy fats, healthy carbohydrates, iron, potassium, calcium, magnesium, Vitamin A, and fiber. Making this soup good for the heart, bones, skin, eyes, blood sugar, blood pressure, brain, and muscle. The fiber is good for weight management also.

This is easy to freeze and pull out for dinner when you don't feel like cooking. It is often made with ham, but you don't need ham for it to taste delicious. Ham adds saturated fat not to mention that the ham alone costs more than all the ingredients combined.

How to Prepare (10 minutes prep time, 30-45 minutes cook time)

You will need: *split peas, potatoes, onions, carrots, garlic cloves, salt, pepper*

1. Place 1 cup of well-rinsed split peas for 1-2 people in a pot with 3-4 cups of water (for a family of 4, use 2 cups of split peas and 4 cups of water).
2. Add 1 large chopped potato, 1 large chopped carrot, 1 large onion, and 3-5 cloves of minced garlic to the pot with the split peas (double ingredients for a family of 4).
3. Add salt and pepper.
4. **Optional step:** Add garlic powder and onion powder to taste.
5. Allow to cook until all ingredients are soft/to the desired consistency (about 30 minutes).
6. Add additional water if necessary.

*Enjoy with salad or crackers.

Nutrition note: **Vitamin B12** is necessary for our bodies to be able to make blood cells and give us energy. Unfortunately, plant-based foods are lacking in this important nutrient. This B12 stays in the body for a while for most of us because it is constantly "recycled";

however, if you choose a vegan diet, it is important to take a B12 supplement over time. If you are a vegetarian, B12 comes from dairy products and eggs. The B12 comes from meat/poultry/fish if you eat meat.

Hearty Lentil Soup
$2.00/serving

Lentils are very versatile and are great for breakfast, lunch, or dinner. And at $2.00 a bag (or 10-14 servings), they don't get any more affordable. They are filled with fiber, protein, healthy carbohydrates, iron, potassium, and more, making them good for growing healthy gut bacteria (part of the microbiome), immune system, blood pressure, blood sugar levels, weight maintenance, digestion, and energy levels.

There are several ways to prepare lentils. Lentil soup, lentils and rice, and lentil patties are my favorite ways to eat them, but you can make lentil salad, lentil curry, lentil meatballs, tacos, lentil loaves, and more. I encourage you to look up recipes for lentils made in different ways. You will not get bored with them.

Lentils come in many forms. Red lentils cook quickly, become mushy, have a milder taste, and are great for soups and lentil patties. Brown or green lentils cook quickly, although not as fast as red lentils. They also maintain their shape better than red lentils. Brown lentils are also great for soups, as an entrée with rice, or for lentil "meatballs." Black lentils are sturdy and crunchy and great to add to grain bowls.

This soup is a full meal in and of itself. I like it with brown or red lentils, depending on my mood or what I have available.

How to Prepare (5 minutes prep time, 30-40 minutes cook time)

You will need: Your *oil of choice, dried, rinsed, and strained red or brown lentils, minced fresh garlic, chopped onions, chopped carrots,*

chopped celery, crushed tomatoes, water or homemade vegetable stock from Chapter 2, salt, pepper, cumin, cayenne pepper
1. Sauté 1 large onion and a few garlic cloves for 4-6 servings. See Chapter 1 for sautéing onions and garlic.
2. Add 1-2 chopped celery sticks and 1-2 chopped carrots to the onions and garlic and allow to soften.
3. Add about 3-4 cups of water/stock, 1 small can of crushed tomatoes, 1.5 cups of lentils, and spices, and bring to a boil.
4. Once it boils, turn the heat down and allow it to simmer for about 30-40 minutes.
    a. I turn the heat off and let it sit for another 30 minutes to allow the flavors to meld together. This also tastes better on the second day.

*When serving, add a tablespoon or two of Greek yogurt or sour cream and fresh herbs to top it off. Enjoy with a salad or crackers.

Lentils and Rice
$1.50/serving

Here is a simple lentil meal that I think your palate will enjoy. I use brown lentils for this.

How to Prepare (5 minutes prep time, 30 minutes cook time)
You will need: *your oil of choice, lentils, brown rice (or quinoa), chopped onions, minced garlic, salt, pepper*
1. Prepare 1 cup of lentils per the instructions on the package (use 2 cups for a family of 4).
2. Prepare ½ cup of rice (or quinoa) per the instructions on the package (use 1 cup for a family of 4).
3. While the lentils and rice are cooking, sauté one small onion and several garlic cloves using the instructions in Chapter 1.
4. Add salt and pepper. Experiment with other spices if you'd like.

5. When the lentils are done, drain them and mix them with the sauteed onions and garlic.
6. When the rice is done, add it to the plate, and place lentils on top.

*Serve with steamed broccoli or your favorite steamed vegetable mentioned in Chapter 1.

Vegetarian Chili
$2.00/serving

If you master one thing to cook, chili is a great meal to choose. It is easy to make, delicious, and affordable. You can make big batches and freeze leftovers, and everybody loves it. This is also a meal that you can prepare with your children. You can even allow them to choose some of the ingredients.

We already went over the benefits of beans in Chapter 1, so we won't rehash that here. Let us dig right in.

How to Prepare (5 minutes prep time, 30-60 minutes cook time)

You will need: *kidney beans, chopped onions, chopped bell peppers, 1 can of crushed tomatoes, fresh garlic, water/vegetable stock, chili powder, cumin, cayenne pepper, salt, pepper*

1. Cook dried beans according to package instructions or see Chapter 1. Use an entire 16-ounce bag for a family of four. For $2.00 more, you can use canned/boxed beans instead.
2. While the beans are cooking, sauté 1 large onion, 3-5 chopped cloves of garlic, and 1 medium green bell pepper (use red for a sweeter taste) until the vegetables are soft.
3. **Optional step:** Add carrots or sweet potatoes.
4. Add the vegetable stock or water, crushed tomatoes, chili powder, cumin, cayenne pepper, salt, and pepper to sauteed veggies and mix (See Chapter 1 for guidance on spice quantities.).
5. Add the beans and bring to a boil.

6. Bring the heat down to a simmer.
7. **Optional step:** For thicker chili, add a tablespoon of cornstarch and stir.
8. **Optional step:** For a richer depth of flavor, add a tablespoon or two of cacao powder and stir.
9. Adjust spices to taste; use garlic powder if the 5 cloves of fresh garlic are not enough. (What can I say? I love garlic).
10. Allow to simmer for 20-30 minutes, stirring occasionally.
11. Pour into a bowl and top with your favorite garnish (Greek yogurt, sour cream, avocado, chopped cilantro or chives, cheddar cheese, chopped green onions are all fair game).

> This is also great for the crockpot/slow cooker. Simply put all the ingredients in the pot, turn it on, go to work, and let it cook for 8 hours. It will be done by the time you get home. Adjust spices to taste. See Chapter 1 for more information on using a slow cooker.

*Enjoy with salad, crackers, or cornbread.

Vegetarian Spaghetti
$1.25/serving

Who says you need to make spaghetti sauce from scratch when you have jarred tomato sauces that just need a little bit of help? Most jarred sauces are made with natural ingredients. The biggest thing to look out for is sodium content because some brands can get out of hand. Also, try to find sauce in glass jars to avoid plastic in your food.

For protein, I use lentil or chickpea pasta which has about 12-15 grams of protein per serving. However, you can add whatever protein source you prefer. Some add tofu, whole lentils, or ground turkey. You will not miss the meat in this. The key is the chunky vegetables and lots and lots of hearty herbs/spices. I grow my own herbs, so I throw a ton in my sauce without worrying about the cost.

How to Prepare (10 minutes prep time, 30 minutes cook time)

You will need: *chopped onion, chopped garlic, chopped bell pepper, chopped mushrooms, jarred spaghetti sauce, dried oregano, garlic powder, dried or fresh basil, black pepper, red pepper flakes, honey*

1. Prepare pasta according to the package instructions (use 8 ounces for 4 servings, 16 ounces for 8 servings).
2. Sauté one large onion and several garlic cloves using the instructions in Chapter 1.
3. Add 1 small chopped red or green bell pepper and 6-10 chopped cremini mushrooms and sauté 5–7 minutes until everything is soft.
4. **Optional step:** Add chopped spinach, shredded carrots, or other veggies.
5. Add a 24-ounce jar of tomato or spaghetti sauce and mix.
6. Add lots of dried oregano, garlic powder, at least ¼ cup chopped fresh basil, and 1-2 tablespoons of honey, salt, pepper, and red pepper flakes to taste.

*Serve with mixed greens and salad dressing or steamed vegetables.

Classic Beans and Rice with Steamed Veggies
$1.50/serving

This meal basically uses the techniques outlined in Chapter 1. Familiarize yourself with these techniques, and you will find most of these meals to be really simple to make. Put the methods all together for this meal, and you get a full meal for about $7.00 for a family of four. Use any type of bean or chickpeas and any type of non-starchy vegetable for something different every night.

How to Prepare (10 minutes prep time, 45-60 minutes cook time)

You will need: *beans, brown rice or quinoa, onions, garlic powder, broccoli or your vegetable of choice, your oil of choice, salt, and pepper*

1. Cook the dried beans. For instructions on cooking dried beans, see Chapter 1 or use canned beans.

2. Cook rice or quinoa according to package instructions.
3. While beans and rice are cooking, steam your vegetable of choice. See Chapter 1 for steaming instructions.
4. While the beans, rice and vegetables are cooking, sauté one medium chopped onion and 3-6 garlic cloves using the instructions in Chapter 1.
5. When the beans are done, strain most of the water, leaving some of the starchy water in the beans (if using canned beans, use some of the starchy water from the rice).
6. Mash some of the beans with the starchy water leaving most of them whole.
7. Add the mashed beans to the sautéed onions and garlic.
8. Add salt, pepper, and more water for a saucier bean.
9. Heat together until the flavors meld (about 5 minutes).
10. For the steamed vegetables, add salt and pepper.

Vegetarian Stuffed Peppers
$3.00/serving

I buy a bag of six organic bell peppers for about $8.00, and we eat them up before my next grocery trip. The bag is cheaper than buying the individual peppers, which can cost $2.00-$3.00 each. I slice them up and eat them raw, use them to make veggie omelets, and sauté them with onions and garlic for a stir fry, tacos, and countless other meals. If I have any whole bell peppers left before my next grocery trip, these stuffed bell peppers are a perfect way to use them up.

Bell peppers are a low-carb, low-calorie, high-fiber, high-potassium, and high-vitamin C food. Stuffed peppers, filled with beans, are a delicious and different way to incorporate a powerful non-starchy vegetable (the pepper) and beans into your food routine. Any color bell pepper will do; just know that red, yellow, and orange bell peppers taste sweeter than green bell peppers. My preference is green or red, depending on the mood I am in.

How to Prepare (10 minutes prep time, 30-45 minutes cook time)

You will need: *bell peppers (one per person), kidney beans, brown rice, onions, garlic, cheddar cheese, salt, pepper, chili powder, cumin, red pepper flakes*

1. Preheat oven to 400°F.
2. Cook the rice according to the package instructions (Use ½ cup dry for four people.)
3. Prepare the beans using instructions on the package or use canned beans.
4. Chop the tops of the bell pepper off and remove the seeds. Pop out and discard/compost the stem from the top portion you just cut off. You will be using that top portion of the pepper.
5. **Optional step:** For an even softer roasted bell pepper, blanch the bell peppers by putting them in boiling hot water for 3-5 minutes.
6. Sauté the onions and garlic per instructions in Chapter 1.
7. Add chili powder, cumin, red pepper flakes, salt, and pepper (Again, use the spice guide in Chapter 1 for quantities.).
8. Drain the rice and beans (save some of the starchy water from the beans or rice) and add to the sauteed onions, garlic, and spices.
9. Add a few sprinkles of shredded cheddar cheese to the beans, onions, and garlic and mix until the cheese is melted.
10. Adjust spices and cheese to taste.
11. Stuff the bell peppers with beans and rice mixture.
12. Place stuffed pepper and the bell pepper tops in the oven for 30-45 minutes or until the bell peppers are soft.
13. **Optional step:** Add shredded cheddar cheese to the top of the bell pepper and place in the oven for 2 more minutes.

Vegetable Omelet

$2.00/serving

Omelets are not just for breakfast and brunch. They are a protein-rich and easy way to add vegetables to the diet. This is another easy meal that children can help with. Serve with a salad and the homemade vinaigrette from Chapter 7.

How to prepare (5 minutes prep time, 5-10 minutes cook time)

You will need: *eggs, your oil of choice, onions, salt, pepper, and any of your favorite vegetables, including bell peppers, mushrooms, spinach, jalapeños, etc.*

1. Sauté the vegetables you choose using the instructions in Chapter 1. Use about ¼ cup of each vegetable for an individual serving.
2. Set the sautéed vegetables aside.
3. Using the same hot pan, over medium heat, add ½ tablespoon of oil.
4. Mix 2 eggs in a bowl and whisk the eggs with a fork.
5. Add the eggs to the hot pan and allow them to spread over the entire pan.
6. Allow to cook for about 30 seconds.
7. Spread the sauteed vegetables on top of the eggs.
8. Fold half of the eggs with veggies over the other half with a spatula forming a pocket.
9. Allow to cook throughout for another 2 minutes.
10. Flip and cook for another minute.
11. Add a sprinkle of salt and pepper.
12. Transfer to a plate. If serving more than one person, repeat. Be sure to sauté enough veggies for the number of people you plan to serve.

13. **Optional step:** Add chopped green onions, fresh chives, avocado slices, fresh chopped tomatoes, and/or Tabasco sauce.

Nutrition note: Tabasco sauce is one of the healthiest store-bought hot sauces. It has the least amount of sodium (35 mg per serving) and is made from vinegar, tabasco, peppers, and salt. That's it.

You can also make **homemade hot sauce.** Simply boil several jalapeños or whatever hot peppers you like (make sure you remove the seeds using gloves), chopped carrots, and/or mango in water. Carrots and mangoes help tame the heat. Boil until everything is soft, and place in a blender. Add a pinch of salt and blend. Strain the sauce to thin it out, or enjoy it thick as is.

If you decide to start a garden after reading this book (see chapter 21), I encourage growing spicy hot peppers like jalapeños, serrano peppers if you like to turn up the heat, or habanero peppers if you like foods that leave burn marks in the mouth! They do well in containers and produce high yields. I don't buy spicy peppers in the summer or fall anymore because I get so many. With the extras, I give them away and make hot sauce!

Homemade Vegan Pizza

$1.75/serving

You would be smart to assume that this vegan pizza uses vegan cheese, but that assumption would be wrong. This pizza requires no cheese at all and tastes just as delicious as pizza with cheese. Instead of pizza dough, I use whole-grain tortillas with no gluten, but you can use whatever you'd like. It is an easy way to incorporate vegetables into your food routine, and children and adults love it. Children can also help prepare the pizzas.

My favorite veggies for this pizza (or any pizza) are mushrooms, onions, small, chopped sprinkles of spinach, and jalapeño or serrano peppers. I also love it with fresh basil, an herb that makes all things (well, almost all things) tomato saucy go from tasting great to amazing. Add leaves like basil and spinach two minutes before the pizza is done to prevent them from burning.

Also, allow me to put a plug in for growing a basil plant in your home. It is always fresh, and it grows back easily after you use it up, so you have a seemingly unlimited supply.

How to prepare (5 minutes prep time, 5-10 minutes cook time)

You will need: *tortillas, tomato paste, salt, pepper, your sweetener and oil of choice, oregano, garlic powder, Italian spice, fresh (or dried) basil, your favorite veggies*

1. Heat oven to 400°F
2. In a small bowl, stir together 6-8 ounces of tomato paste, a pinch of salt and black pepper, about 1-2 teaspoons of sweetener (I use honey), and about 1-2 teaspoons of oil (I use olive oil) for four 8-inch pizzas.
3. Add water ounce by ounce until it reaches your desired consistency.
4. Add 1-2 teaspoons of the oregano, garlic powder, and Italian spices. If using dried basil, add it now.
5. Arrange tortillas/dough onto baking sheets.
6. Spread the tomato sauce onto each tortilla, leaving about ½ inch at the edges.
7. Layer your favorite vegetable slices on top of the sauce.
8. Bake for 10 minutes until veggies are soft on the inside and crispy on the outside.
    a. Add fresh basil or spinach 2 minutes before the pizza is done and bake the remaining 2 minutes.

*You can also use this as a base. Add cheese or anything else you'd like, but these pizzas taste delicious as they are.

Using Millet Instead of Rice
$0.35/serving ($6.00/16-ounce package)

If you are tired of rice and want to try something different, millet is another very affordable gluten-free grain that you might enjoy. It adds a crunchy bite to your meals or can be made into a filling breakfast porridge. You can add peanut butter to plain millet and make little energy balls.

Like rice, you can season it or just let it take on the flavor of the food you serve. It has more protein and fiber than rice, making it a filling grain that you will only need a small amount of to feel satisfied. One cup dry makes about 3.5 cups cooked.

How to Prepare (2 minutes prep time, 30 minutes cook time)
You will need: *millet, water*
1. Put 1 part millet for 2 parts water in a saucepan. I recommend starting with ½ cup of millet and 1 cup of water which yields about 2 cups.
2. Bring water to a boil.
3. Turn the heat down and allow it to simmer for 30 minutes or until the water has been absorbed.
4. Use in place of rice.

*To make millet porridge for breakfast, follow steps 1 – 3. Add spices like cinnamon or nutmeg, vanilla, a pinch of salt, or milk during step one. To make it very creamy, you can blend the final product. Then add raisins, fresh fruit, or a sweetener to top it off.

Using Quinoa Instead of Rice
$0.60/serving ($3.00/8 ounce package)

Quinoa is unique because it is one of the only plant-based foods that is a complete protein. It's also a delicious, fluffy, affordable, naturally gluten-free grain with 5 grams of fiber per serving, iron, and potassium. Use it in place of rice for an extra nutrient boost. One cup dry makes about 4 cups cooked. Follow the instructions on the packages or use the instructions below.

How to Prepare (2 minutes prep time, 30 minutes cook time)

You will need: *Quinoa and water*
1. Boil 2 cups of water.
2. Add one cup of quinoa and return it to a boil.
3. Reduce heat to medium and cover.
4. Simmer until water is absorbed (10-15 minutes).
5. Remove from heat and fluff.
6. Allow to stand for 10-15 minutes.

Classic Grain Bowl

$3.00/serving

This meal works well for breakfast, lunch, or dinner and is another way to add several veggies to your food routine. You just need a grain like rice, millet, or quinoa, 2-3 of your favorite vegetables, beans or other protein, and a sauce. This is also a great place to put those pickled veggies we mentioned in the first chapter and get those probiotics that create a healthy microbiome in the gut. It is also great to get children involved in making this meal.

How to Prepare (5 minutes prep time, 20 minutes cook time)

You will need: *Quinoa, onions, broccoli, shredded carrots, sliced cucumbers, and/or your favorite veggies, chickpeas (or your favorite protein), olive oil, vinegar*
1. Prepare the quinoa per the package instructions or see the previous page. Use ¼ cup dry for one serving.
2. Sauté, roast, or steam the veggies you choose. Use ½ cup of each per serving.
3. **Optional step:** Chop up or slice a sweet potato, roast, and add to your bowl.
4. Slice the cucumber and shred the carrots. Use the amount that feels right to you per serving.

5. Prepare the chickpeas per package instructions or use rinse canned versions. Use the amount that feels right to you per serving.
6. Use the homemade vinaigrette recipe from Chapter 7 or choose a store-bought sauce.
7. Build your bowl.
8. **Optional step:** Add hummus, avocado, and homemade pickled veggies.

*There are a million ways to create a grain bowl. Find some online recipes or experiment yourself. You can even try to imitate popular food chains like Cava and Mezeh restaurants.

* * *

We have multiple meals that we can prepare or cook at home. Let us now talk about eating out on a budget.

CHAPTER 9

EATING OUT ON A BUDGET

Everybody loves to eat out occasionally. I mean, who doesn't love the feeling of someone preparing food for you while the only thing you have to do is enjoy the food? There are some things to be aware of when we eat out though:

- ☑ About 71 percent of sodium in our diets comes from prepared and processed foods; five percent is added at the table, and six percent is added while cooking.[22]
- ☑ There might be loads of sugar, salt, unhealthy fat, chemicals, preservatives, dyes, and more in that food.
- ☑ Prepared foods are almost always more expensive than preparing food at home.

Here are some tips for navigating these food pitfalls while saving at the same time:

- ☑ Sometimes, you can find nutrition facts and ingredient information on the restaurant's website. You may still choose the food you were planning to eat, but at least you know what is in it.
- ☑ If you don't want to look up this information, go for the simple meals like:
    - Salads (They cost just as much as the sandwiches/meals now.)

- Soups made mostly with vegetables, beans, or lentils
- Beans, rice, and vegetables
- The choice of three vegetarian sides
- Vegetarian sushi rolls
- Seasoned roasted, baked, or grilled tofu, fish, or poultry
- ☑ Forget the appetizer and the dessert. Saves money and calories.
- ☑ Save half of your meal for the next day. Ask the waiter for a to-go box at the beginning of the meal and save the other half for later. You get dinner/lunch for two days for the price of one.
- ☑ Choose the free filtered tap water option to save calories and money.
- ☑ Order the smallest size or order from the children's menu.
- ☑ For fast-food restaurants, order the sandwich without the meal. Most sandwiches are calorie-wise, meals all their own.
- ☑ For fast-food restaurants, bring your own beverage. If you are not into that, most restaurants will give you a cup for free water or provide bottled water for the same price as the sweetened drink.

Choosing the Vegetarian Option

You can often swap meat options with vegetarian options; beans, tofu, and avocado are often substitute offerings depending on the dish. Minus the bioengineered meats, vegetarian options are usually healthier and lower in cost, calories, and saturated fat.

Several fast-food places are better at providing healthier vegetarian options at a lower price. Watch out for those fast-food restaurants and burger joints that try to charge more. Here are some examples of vegetarian options, usually at a reduced cost:

- Salads
- Tacos/burritos

- Subs
- Wraps
- Bowls
- Pasta dishes

Speaking of pasta, some restaurants offer zoodles as a replacement. Zoodles are noodles made with zucchini and are one of the healthiest alternatives to pasta. You can also make zoodles at home with a spiralizer, which costs between $10.00-$50.00.

After making a zoodle recipe for one of my classes, a student told me at the next class that she bought a spiralizer and put a bunch of zucchini noodles in a large container. Her children started eating them, and now, they love making and using them for various recipes. You can also use a spiralizer for beets, carrots, parsnips, sweet potatoes, and so much more.

Caution: Vegan or Vegetarian Does Not Always Mean Healthy

I went to a vegan establishment with a friend. While we were in line, he mentioned that he felt good that he was doing something healthy for his body. I knew that the food was mostly made from meat substitutes, white bread, sauces, and French fries. I told him that he is doing good for the planet and animals, but maybe not so much for his body.

Surprised, he asked if it was better than red meat or pork. I told him that it remains to be seen because there is no research on the long-term effect of these meat substitutes. Some meat substitutes have similar amounts of saturated fat and more sodium than beef, but they don't have any cholesterol. The alternatives don't have hormones and antibiotics either. Despite that, there is a chance that they are not better alternatives to actual meat, given that they are highly processed and contain several additives.

> Lay low on the meat substitutes since the jury is still out on their health benefits.

Also, your body knows how to process beef and pork. The body isn't as efficient at processing new food innovations. In fact, as is the case with trans fats mentioned in Chapter 15, sometimes it can be more harmful to our body/health than the product it is trying to mimic. For now, then, if you do choose to eat these foods, know that you are doing something good for animals and the environment, but not so much for your health.

Meat Alternatives vs. Veggie Burger

You might see two options on the menu: the Meat Substitute Burger or the Veggie Burger. The veggie burger is the better option for health unless you have an allergy or sensitivity to any of the ingredients in the burger. The veggie burger is usually made with nutrient-rich plant-based options like black beans, vegetables, and quinoa. The meat substitute is made with a genetically engineered, lab-grown product and additives.

Choosing Frozen Foods/Meals

Healthy frozen meals (including the ones with "healthy" in the name) can be hard to come by. But there are a few frozen dinner options that don't cost an arm and a leg and are better alternatives to the cheesy beef lasagna and other dinners that have a lot of saturated fat, chemical-laden meats, additives, and preservatives.

Below are a few frozen meal recommendations, but always check the nutrition facts and ingredients label when choosing your meals using the tips from chapter 13.

Frozen Meals Under $15 for a Family of 2-4

Entrées:
- Black bean/vegetable burgers (not the meat substitutes)
- Turkey or chicken burgers
- Frozen stir-fry dinners
- Beans, vegetables, and rice dinners
- Stuffed pepper dinners
- Grain bowls
- Vegetable cauliflower crust pizzas
- Frozen chicken breast cutlets and veggies
- Frozen grilled chicken breast strips/cubes and veggies
- Chicken fajitas with onions and peppers

Frozen Sides:
- Frozen French fries or sweet potato fries
- Frozen vegetables (including red and sweet potatoes)
- Rice with mixed vegetables
- Cauliflower rice

There is still a stigma attached to people (women in particular) who don't cook at home. But if you have the funds and can find healthy prepared foods without all the sodium and preservatives, then go for it and forget what others say.

This book is not about reinforcing that stigma. I promote food preparation at home because it is hard to find healthy (per our definition) prepared foods, even at higher price points. Cooking at home allows us to adjust our tastes to our bodies' needs and wants. It is also more affordable and, therefore, a very useful tool in helping us achieve our health goals within our budgets.

CHAPTER 10

SAMPLE GROCERY LIST AND MENU

Preparing a grocery list can be annoying, but it can save a lot of money. That is why I put together a grocery list and menu to serve as an example of the possibilities. Here are some tips to help shopping go a little easier:

- ☑ Purchase groceries once every two weeks. It saves money and time. Your fruits and vegetables will last if stored well (See Chapter 2 for more on storing produce.).
- ☑ Eat foods that go bad faster first. For example, cucumbers don't last as long as carrots so eat up the cucumbers first.
- ☑ Take a trip to a warehouse once a month to stock up for the month.
- ☑ Look up local food distributions near you and stock up.

Two Week Menu for Family of Four (about $150 or $75 per week)

BREAKFAST	• Egg muffins and clementine oranges • Oatmeal, nuts, and apples • Yogurt and berries
LUNCH	• Open-face tuna sandwich with carrot sticks and cucumber slices • Peanut butter sandwich and apple slices • Salad • Dinner leftovers

DINNER	• Black beans, avocado slices, rice and broccoli • Chickpeas, onions, rice, and kale salad • Roasted chicken, quinoa, garlic spinach • Frozen dinner of choice
SNACKS/ DESSERTS	• Banana • Pineapples • Zucchini sticks and salad dressing • Applesauce • Berries and whipped cream • Peanuts • Crackers and cheese • Popcorn • Your favorite snack chip
DRINKS	• Water • 100% Juice

FOOD ITEM	PRICE
Fruit ($38.00)	
1 bag of avocados (4 count)	$5.00
1 bag of apples (5 pounds)*	$7.00
1 bag of clementines (5 pounds)	$7.00
16 bananas	$5.00
2 bags of frozen berries (16 ounces each)	$8.00
2 large fresh pineapples	$6.00
Vegetables ($26.00)	
2 bulbs of fresh garlic	$1.00
1 bag of onions (3 pounds)*	$3.00
2 broccoli crowns (4 pounds)	$4.00
11-ounce container of spinach	$5.00
2 bunches of kale	$4.00
1 bag of baby carrots (3 pounds)*	$3.00
4 cucumbers	$3.00
3 large zucchinis	$3.00
Protein ($39.00)	
16-ounce bag of chickpeas, dried*	$2.00
16-ounce bag of black beans, dried*	$2.00
1 bag of walnuts or pecans (16 ounces)	$6.00
1 jar of peanuts (16 ounces)*	$3.00
3 5-ounce cans of tuna fish*	$6.00
1 whole roasted chicken	$8.00

FOOD ITEM	PRICE
2 cartons of eggs (12 count)	$8.00
A 32-ounce container of plain yogurt	$4.00
Grains ($23.00)	
1 18-ounce container of oatmeal*	$4.00
1 5-pound bag of rice*	$4.00
1 16-ounce bag of quinoa*	$5.00
2 bags of popcorn	$6.00
1 loaf of bread*	$4.00
Other ($32.00)	
4 frozen dinners	$16.00
1 8-ounce block of cheese*	$3.00
Salad dressing	$4.00
1 bag of your favorite snack chip	$3.00
2 ½-gallon-cartons of 100% juice*	$6.00

*Signifies a food that you will be likely to find at a food pantry/food distribution or government program mentioned in Chapter 21.

Your healthy food arsenal is now filled with affordable drinks, snacks, breakfast, lunch, dinner, and ideas for eating out. I found that having this information is necessary but not always sufficient to fully arm ourselves with what we need to make the best food choices for our health.

Many of my students think they are making healthy choices because of an article they read or an advertisement they saw. When they come to my class, they realize that may not be the case and ask lots of questions about nutrition. And that is why I present to you part two…THE KNOWLEDGE.

PART 2
THE KNOWLEDGE
NUTRITION BASICS

CHAPTER 11

WHY DO YOU WANT TO BE HEALTHY?

Part one established that healthy eating can be affordable. You are now about to learn the fundamentals of nutrition that will give you the confidence you need to make an informed choice about your food.

If a healthy diet is your goal, knowing what a healthy choice looks like is important. Knowing what is healthy can get confusing with all the claims on packaged and prepared foods. For example, just because a product says "high in protein," "plant-based," or "contains whole grains," that does not make it a healthy food. We'll sort through all of this. But first, here is a reminder of the definitions that you will need for this chapter:

- ☑ Diet = what you eat in a day (not a strict food regimen where foods are eliminated).
- ☑ Processed foods = foods that are mostly made from factory-made additives (like artificial colors, stabilizers, artificial sweeteners, and preservatives) and/or natural foods stripped of their nutrition (like sugar, flour, and oils). They also include hot dogs, sodas, shelf-stable cookies, etc.
- ☑ Healthy foods = foods that contain the nutrients needed for optimal health and do no harm.

"Do no harm" is the key here. For example, would beef be considered healthy? It is high in protein and other nutrients important for optimal health, like iron. However, there is evidence to suggest that consuming beef is correlated with a higher risk of heart disease and several cancers (including breast, colon, and more)[23]. I, therefore, would not include beef of any kind as a healthy food because of the potential for harm.

Focus on Adding Foods, Not Subtracting Them

Healthy eating is not always about eliminating foods but about incorporating healthy foods into your everyday life. In fact, the more emphasis you put on trying to eliminate foods from your diet, the less mental energy you have to choose healthy foods. The more you say, "I can't eat xyz,"–the chances are you are going to want to eat it. Instead, focus on and fill up on the healthy foods you want to eat. The unhealthy foods you don't want to eat will become less and less desirable over time as your taste readjusts. Something like adding one piece of fruit or vegetable daily may seem like a small step, but remember, small steps make a big difference.

> Remember, a "healthy diet" is not about restriction, but instead about adding more healthy options that promote optimal health and do not cause harm.

Know Your Why

As is true with any goal, it is important to know your reason for wanting to achieve that goal and to regularly remind yourself of that reason. Especially when the going gets tough. I have several reasons that I remind myself of regularly. First, I want to be able to contribute what I know I can contribute to the world, and I remember I can't contribute without my physical, emotional, and mental health. Second, I have a scary eye condition that I used to take medication for; however, the medicines had horrible side effects, and I was losing my vision slowly but surely. I figured out that I can control my condition with my diet, and I remind myself of that when I choose what I am going to eat. Not that I don't forget or splurge sometimes (ok, many times), but having those reasons helps keep me on track for those times when I fall off. And I try not to beat myself up when I fall off track (something we will discuss more in chapter 19). I just get back on the train and ride.

> Know your reason for wanting to achieve a healthy diet and write it down. Remember that reason when choosing your food.

There is no right or wrong "reason" to want to eat healthily. I would only caution against eating a healthy diet because someone else told you to do it or because people/society are pressuring you. Be clear about what YOU want and why YOU want it. Then write it down and put it in a place where you will be reminded of it. There is a space below for you to write your reasons down. Or write it in a journal.

* * *

What is your reason(s) for choosing healthy?

1. _____
_____

2. _____
_____

3. _____
_____

4. _____
_____

Next, Decide What Your Commitment Is Going to Be

I will also recommend that you decide what your commitment will be and write it down. Commitment, in this instance, is deciding how much of your time and resources you are going to put into achieving your health goals (to be distinguished from setting health goals themselves). There is no commitment level too big or too small. Just make sure it is realistic for you and that you decide to put some effort toward it. Here are a few examples of commitments:

- ☑ I commit $10.00 more of my weekly food budget to healthy foods.
- ☑ I commit 15 minutes to achieving my health goals at the beginning of the week.
- ☑ I dedicate one shelf in my food pantry/fridge for healthy foods.
- ☑ I dedicate one section of my countertop space to healthy foods.

The powerful thing about deciding what your commitment will be and writing it down is that if you don't stick to that commitment, you have a reference point to return to. Didn't hit the mark today? That's ok, start over the next day. Chapter 19 reveals a little bit about the power behind giving yourself grace. So, dropping the ball is fine. Go ahead and tell yourself that it's ok. Just have something concrete to go back to if/when you do.

What is your commitment(s)?

1. _____

_____

2. _____
   _____

3. _____
   _____

4. _____
   _____

Graduate to Your Next Commitment

Part of setting goals is to set a new goal once you achieve your initial goal. It's the same process when it comes to commitments. Once you have committed to spending an extra $5.00 a week on healthy food, see if you have space to expand your commitment level further. Perhaps $7.00 or $10.00 a week is your next commitment level. These might seem like small numbers but be patient; your commitment levels will grow over time.

Shift the Way You Think About Healthy Foods

Recall that choosing healthy options is not always more expensive, and healthy foods are not always "nasty." Let's go back to the beef example. On average, one serving of beef (3-4 ounces) costs about $1.50 per serving. Dried beans cost about $0.30 per serving (5-6 ounces cooked). So, it is more expensive to eat something that can increase your risk for heart disease and cancer.

Healthy food is also delicious. You are likely one or two herbs or spices away from a delicious meal. Since many of our tastes have been heavily shaped by the processed food industry, some vegetables like kale and collards may be difficult to eat plain, but if you add some healthy oils, herbs, and spices, they are delicious and still very healthy.

Mindset Reset
Healthy food is affordable and tastes delicious.

If you come into the gate thinking, "It's too expensive" and "It doesn't taste good," that is another battle you must overcome.

Let's review!

- ☑ Learning the basics will give us the confidence to make healthy choices.
- ☑ Taking things step by step will increase our likelihood of achieving our health goals over the long term.
- ☑ Focusing on eating the healthy foods we want, not the foods we are trying to eliminate, shifts our energy in a positive direction.
- ☑ Knowing our "reason" will be a motivating force.
- ☑ Deciding what our commitment will be will help us stay on track.
- ☑ Resetting our mindset about healthy eating removes a barrier to success.

Now that we have a new mindset and concrete actions that can set us up for success, let us arm ourselves with some knowledge to help us make informed choices about what we put in our bodies.

CHAPTER 12

CALORIES

This chapter provides a foundation for understanding the components of the food we eat. It will make things like understanding nutrition facts labels and reading the ingredients list less confusing so you can make a more informed choice about your food. Let's start with one of the most talked about measures of food…calories.

What Are Calories?

Calories are a way to measure the energy that we receive from food. That energy is used for body functions like movement, breathing, digestion, thinking, organ function (e.g., brain, heart, lungs, liver, etc.), and much more. The energy we don't use for these functions is mostly stored in the body as fat.

Where do Calories Come From?

We receive calories from the following sources:
- Carbohydrates
- Fats
- Protein
- Alcohol

> Water does not have any calories/energy. Instead, it is the thing that allows us to access the energy we get from carbohydrates, fats, and proteins.

Carbohydrates, fats, and protein are very important nutrients essential to human life. Alcohol is not an essential nutrient, although many of us get several of our calories from alcohol. Water, while it is essential to life, has zero calories.

Each of these calorie sources (carbohydrates, fats, proteins, and alcohol) is measured in grams, and each gram contains a specific number of calories.

- 1 gram of carbohydrates has about 4 calories.
- 1 gram of protein has about 4 calories.
- 1 gram of fat has about 9 calories.
- 1 gram of alcohol has about 7 calories.

How to Calculate the Number of Calories from Different Nutrients?

To calculate the number of calories that come from any of these nutrients (i.e., carbs, protein, fat, alcohol), multiply the number of grams in the food (which can be found on the package) by the number of calories found in 1 gram.

Example:
A food with 5 grams of carbohydrates and
5 grams of fat has 65 total calories.

5 grams carbohydrates × 4 calories per gram = 20 calories
5 grams fats × 9 calories per gram = 45 calories
Total = 65 calories

How Many Calories Should I be Eating?

It depends on multiple factors. We all need a certain amount of carbohydrates, protein, and fats (see chapters 14-16) just to live.

This is based on height, weight, and genetics. But then we need more calories to fuel our everyday physical activities, whether it's going to work or running a marathon. Obviously, running a marathon is going to require more calories than someone who sits at a desk for most of the day at work.

Because of these variables and more, it is difficult to determine an individual's exact caloric (or energy) needs. However, we can get an idea with the basal metabolic rate or BMR.

What Is the Basal Metabolic Rate (BMR)?

The basal metabolic rate (BMR) is an estimate of the number of calories/energy we need to maintain all our bodily functions (e.g., digestion, breathing, thinking, etc.) and daily functions (exercise, working, etc.) for each day.

If we eat more calories than we need, the body will store the extra energy, mostly as fat. If we eat fewer calories than we need, the body will pull energy from our fat stores to make up the deficit. People often use their BMR to help them with weight management. It is useful for us to be aware of how much energy our bodies need.

Our BMR is a useful number, but it is not a perfect number. Use it as a reference point to work from. Then also, pay attention to how your body responds to different quantities of food.

Information You Need to Calculate Your BMR:
- Height
- Weight
- Age
- Physical activity levels

Below is the formula for calculating one's BMR. The formula is pretty complex, so to get around all of the math, you can go online and search "BMR calculator" and let the internet do the work for you.

How to Calculate Your BMR?

BMR for Men
= 66.47 + (13.75 x weight [kg]) + (5.003 x size [cm])
− (6.755 x age [years])

BMR for Women
= 655.1 + (9.563 x weight [kg]) + (1.85 x size [cm])
− (4.676 x age [years])

For example, The BMR for a 50-year-old, 200-pound, 5'8 male who does not exercise would be. 2,090 calories.

> A BMR of 2,090 means that if he consumes less than 2,090 calories, he will use up some of his fat stores. If he consumes more than 2,090 calories, he will store the extra energy/calories as fat. If he consumes that amount, he will not lose or store any fat.

I am not a proponent of calorie counting; however, we tend to consume to the point of harm. Much of that overconsumption is a result of the increasing sizes of our portions over the years. Everything from bagels to bottled soda pop comes in much larger sizes than it did years ago. Knowing how many calories we actually need can bring us back to consuming levels right for our bodies and health.

Calories and Aging

Research suggests that eating more calories than we need ages us faster and that reducing our caloric intake while optimizing nutrition can reduce the effects of aging.[24] When we eat what we need, we save money because we don't have to buy as much food. We also save because we experience less illness and, therefore, have less need for medications and medical procedures.

This does not mean that we should starve ourselves, just that we should pay attention to what our body needs, whether it is 1,500 calories a day or 2,500 calories a day.

Where Should My Calories Come From?

Calories come from three types of nutrients: carbohydrates, fats, and protein. Recall that alcohol is not essential for life, even though many of us consume many of our calories from alcohol. Table 12.1 provides the USDA recommendation for the percentage of calories that should come from each nutrient.

— TABLE 12.1 —
RECOMMENDED QUANTITIES OF CARBOHYDRATES, FAT, AND PROTEIN PER DAY

	ACCEPTABLE MACRONUTRIENT DISTRIBUTION RANGES (AMDR)[25]	E.G., CALORIES FOR SOMEONE WHO REQUIRES 1,500 CALORIES PER DAY WOULD BE
Carbohydrates	45-65%	675-975
Fat	20-35%	300-525
Protein	10-35%	150-525

*While we get calories from alcohol, it is not a nutrient necessary for life, so it is omitted here.

Some fad diets grossly distort these numbers. One is a high-fat, low-carbohydrate diet, where the percentage of fat and protein is much higher than the carbohydrate percentage. Another is a low-fat fad diet, which brings the fat percentage down to seemingly zero. These fad diets are usually designed for weight loss, not optimal health, and they are not sustainable.

> All of these numbers (and the numbers that are to come) are good to have as a guide, but do not have the final say. Your body does. Pay attention to your body and how it responds to different foods and food quantities, even whole foods.

Are All Calories the Same?

A better question is what comes along with that calorie? What comes along with that particular carbohydrate, fat, or protein? Do fiber, vitamins, and minerals surround it, and is it in its natural form, as is the case with whole foods? Or has it been extracted from its original source, as is the case with white sugar and other refined grains like white flour (see Chapter 14)?

Below are two charts that provide a rough sense of what happens to blood sugar for the same type of carbohydrate in different forms (whole vs. refined). The refined form (left chart) spikes blood sugar almost immediately and then causes a crash. You know when you get that rush of energy and then feel tired minutes later after eating that muffin. 100% whole grains (right chart) gradually raise blood sugar because they have fiber, fat, and protein. Fiber, fat, and protein slow down the processing of the sugar so that it doesn't spike. Whole grains, therefore, give you longer-lasting energy without the crash. This extra support from the fiber, fat, and protein also means that whole grains fill us up faster and that we are less likely to eat as much.

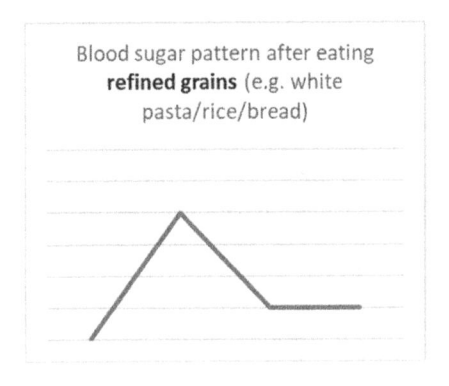

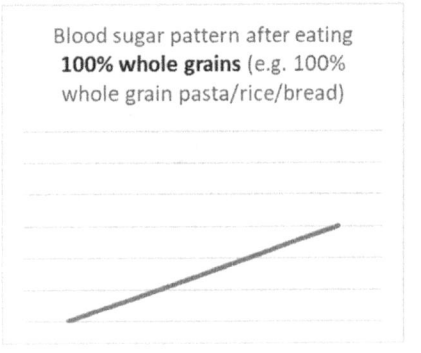

Calories from whole foods are in an environment that will allows us to maximize health benefits best.

Blood sugar pattern after eating **refined grains** (e.g. white pasta/rice/bread)

Blood sugar pattern after eating **100% whole grains** (e.g. 100% whole grain pasta/rice/bread)

Carbohydrates demonstrate how different calories from the same nutrient in different environments can affect the body in different ways. In that sense, a calorie is still a calorie; it just acts differently.

I'd like to reemphasize that you pay attention to how certain foods impact your body and mood. Some people do better with more carbohydrates, and some do better with less. It is the same with whole proteins and healthy fats. Chapters 14-16 will provide more information on the healthiest carbs, fats, and proteins so you can make even better health choices. Eating what is right for your body will help you burn calories more efficiently. Speaking of burning calories efficiently, let's talk about metabolism.

What Is Metabolism?

Metabolism is the process our bodies use to convert calories into energy. As we discovered with calories, this energy is used for everyday functions like breathing and moving. BMR is one aspect of metabolism that gives us a sense of how much energy we need to live. Let's take things a little further to understand metabolism better.

Think of your body as a cozy wood-burning fire. The fire is blue, shy, small, and slowly burns wood when your metabolism is low. When your metabolism is high, the fire is red, big, bold, and quickly burns wood. The more you feed the fire (body) the right type of materials (whole foods and exercise), the better you can maintain that fire and metabolize your food efficiently.

There is scientific evidence to suggest that some foods can increase metabolism. Here are a few of those foods:
- Ginger[26]
- Turmeric[27]
- Cayenne pepper[28]
- Green tea[29]

Exercise and proper sleep can also help to increase metabolism.[30,31] Genetics also plays a major role in how our bodies burn energy, but it is outside of our control, and we want to focus on what we can control.

Determining the Number of Calories You Eat in a Day

To help my clients with their journey to a healthier diet, first and foremost, I give them a sense of how many calories they are currently eating. Most are often shocked to learn how much they eat daily.

I ask them to record what they eat on two to three typical days. Including a weekday and a weekend day is important. I prompt them for meals, snacks, drinks, and condiments (Don't forget those calorie-laden condiments.). Table 12.2 is the form I ask them to fill out. If you are interested in tracking your own food intake, make copies of this form and fill it out as you go throughout the day.

I normally calculate the total number of calories for the individual, but you can do it yourself. To find out the number of calories in each food, drink, or condiment, use the following resources:

- ☑ The nutrition facts label. You can find the information on most large grocery store websites.
- ☑ Visit the restaurant/food company website.
- ☑ Do an internet search.
- ☑ Purchase a calorie-counting app. There aren't too many free apps anymore. However, the USDA's FoodData Central website (https://fdc.nal.usda.gov/) is a free alternative to purchasing an app, albeit not as user-friendly.

Remember to record the correct portion sizes. Also, calculate the calories according to how much you actually eat, not the number on the package. For example, you may eat two cups of cereal for breakfast, but the label might give you information for one cup. If you eat two cups, multiply the number on the nutrition facts label by two. If you eat three cups, multiply the number by three, etc.

— TABLE 12.2 —
FOOD LOG

TIME	LIST FOOD ITEMS AND PORTION SIZES (CALORIES IN PARENTHESIS) *(INCLUDE MEALS, SNACKS, CONDIMENTS, AND BRAND NAME OR HOMEMADE)*	DRINKS AND PORTION SIZES	APPROXIMATE TOTAL # OF CALORIES *(ADD CALORIES AND PUT HERE)*
Example 8 a.m.	McDowell's egg and cheese sandwich (400 calories) w/ 2 packs mayonnaise (200), 1 pack of salt and pepper (0) 2 hash browns (250), 2 packs ketchup (75)	16 oz PJ's coffee (0 calories) 4 packs of sugar (64 calories)	985 calories
6 a.m.			
7 a.m.			
8 a.m.			
9 a.m.			
10 a.m.			
11 a.m.			
Noon			
1 p.m.			
2 p.m.			
3 p.m.			
4 p.m.			
5 p.m.			
6 p.m.			
7 p.m.			
8 p.m.			
9 p.m.			

TIME	LIST FOOD ITEMS AND PORTION SIZES (CALORIES IN PARENTHESIS) *(INCLUDE MEALS, SNACKS, CONDIMENTS, AND BRAND NAME OR HOMEMADE)*	DRINKS AND PORTION SIZES	APPROXIMATE TOTAL # OF CALORIES *(ADD CALORIES AND PUT HERE)*
10 p.m.			
11 p.m.			
Midnight			
1 a.m.			
2 a.m.			
3 a.m.			
4 a.m.			
5 a.m.			

We now know that calories are a way to measure the energy we consume. That energy is used to maintain life, as things like movement, sleeping, and breathing all require energy. The sources of this energy come in the form of fats, proteins, and carbohydrates (and alcohol). The following chapters will help us distinguish the best sources of calories. But first, let us determine the quantity of calories and other nutrients that are in the foods we eat using the nutrition facts label and ingredients list.

CHAPTER 13

DECODING THE MYSTERIES OF THE NUTRITION FACTS LABEL AND INGREDIENTS LIST

You've probably seen or used it, but do you know if you are using it correctly? I am talking about the nutrition facts label and the ingredients list on food packages. The nutrition facts label provides the quantity of specific nutrients in our foods. The ingredients list provides, as you might imagine, the ingredients. The Food and Drug Administration (FDA) requires that food manufacturers include this information on their packaged foods.

It can get confusing because they pack lots of useful information into a little bit of space. This chapter will help you decode these labels and lists so that you can gain the confidence you need to make a healthy choice just by looking at the package.

The Ingredients List

Before looking at the nutrition facts label, I look at the ingredients list. Per the FDA, "The ingredient list on a food label is the listing of each ingredient in descending order of predominance."[32]

Figure 1, for example, has more enriched flour than any other ingredient because it is listed first. After enriched flour, sugar is the most prominent ingredient. The ingredients in parenthesis are the contents of the enriched flour.

After sugar, partially hydrogenated cottonseed oil is the next prominent ingredient, and so on. As you go down the list, we can tell that there are fewer mono- and diglycerides than any other ingredient because they are listed last. (Mono- and diglycerides are emulsifiers that prevent the separation of water and oil.)

Nutrition Facts

Ingredients: Enriched flour (wheat flour, malted barley, niacin, reduced iron, thiamin mononitrate, riboflavin, folic acid), sugar, partially hydrogenated cottonseed oil, high fructose corn syrup, whey (milk), eggs, vanilla, natural and artificial flavoring, salt, leavening (sodium acid pyrophosphate, monocalcium phosphate), lecithin (soy), mono- and diglycerides.

Any Cookie Company
College Park, MD 20740

Figure 1. Sample Ingredients List[33]

Do you think the food represented in Figure 1 would qualify as healthy food per our definition? (Definition reminder; Healthy foods = foods that contain the nutrients needed for optimal health and do no harm.)

In some cases, you can decide if the food is healthy or not right off the bat. In this case, for example, you would be eating mostly flour and sugar. So, without looking at anything else, this would not be considered a healthy food. But what if the first ingredients are healthy ingredients, does that mean it is healthy? Not necessarily, because what else is in there?

Since so many of our packaged foods have additives, refined, and artificial ingredients, a good general rule is that if the product has ingredients you don't recognize, even if it is listed in the middle or last on the list, you might want to put it back on the shelf. It doesn't matter how many health claims they try to make on the front of the package. Companies use buzzwords like "protein," "100% whole grain," "plant-based," or "organic" to try and convince us that their product is healthy. Having these qualities does not make the product healthy. You need to see what ingredients are in the food before making that determination.

> The ingredients list should have ingredients that you recognize. If it does not, and you are looking for a healthy choice, put it back on the shelf.

On occasion a lesser-known ingredient like ascorbic acid (which is just vitamin C) will appear on the list. However, in a vast majority of cases, the ingredient that you don't recognize will be something that is not healthy for our bodies.

If the product has ingredients you recognize and *know are healthy*, that is a good sign. The next thing to do is look at the nutrition facts label.

The Nutrition Facts Label

The nutrition facts label provides information about the nutrients found in packaged food. See Figure 2 for an example of a nutrition facts label. The numbers on the label are not exact; however, they are still useful because they provide roundabout estimates. We are going to walk through the following components of the label together:

- ☑ Serving Size, Servings Per Container and Calories
- ☑ The nutrient quantity (either in grams or milligrams) for nutrients like carbohydrates, fats, proteins, and several vitamins and minerals
- ☑ The Percent (%) Daily Value

You will need to use a little math for some of this, so get ready!

Nutrition Facts

8 servings per container
Serving size 2/3 cup (55g)

Amount per serving
Calories 230

	% Daily Value*
Total Fat 8g	10%
Saturated Fat 1g	5%
Trans Fat 0g	
Cholesterol 0mg	0%
Sodium 160mg	7%
Total Carbohydrate 37g	13%
Dietary Fiber 4g	14%
Total Sugars 12g	
Includes 10g Added Sugars	20%
Protein 3g	
Vitamin D 2mcg	10%
Calcium 260mg	20%
Iron 8mg	45%
Potassium 240mg	6%

* The % Daily Value (DV) tells you how much a nutrient in a serving of food contributes to a daily diet. 2,000 calories a day is used for general nutrition advice

Figure 2. FDA Nutrition Facts Label Example[34]

Serving Size

Take a second to identify the serving size for the sample frozen lasagna nutrition facts label in Figure 3. Did you find that the serving size is one cup? That serving size is important because all the information that follows pertains to that one cup and that one cup only, not the entire contents of the package.

For example, look on the label, and you will find that one cup of this food item has 280 calories. Therefore, if I were to eat two cups, I'd consume 560 calories. This is true for every other nutrient listed.

The product in Figure 3 also has 9 grams (g) of fat, 35 milligrams (mg) of cholesterol, 15 grams of protein, etc., *per serving*. Doing a little bit of math, this means that two cups of this product would have:

- ☑ 18 grams of fat (9 grams x 2 servings)
- ☑ 70 milligrams of cholesterol (35 milligrams x 2 servings)
- ☑ 30 grams of protein (15 grams x 2 servings)
- ☑ Etc.

Nutrition Facts

1. Serving Information
2. Calories
3. Nutrients
4. Quick Guide to percent Daily Value (%DV)
   - 5% or less is **low**
   - 20% or more is **high**

4 servings per container
Serving size   1 cup (227g)

Amount per serving
Calories 280

	% Daily Value*
Total Fat 9g	12%
Saturated Fat 4.5g	23%
Trans Fat 0g	
Cholesterol 35mg	12%
Sodium 850mg	37%
Total Carbohydrate 34g	12%
Dietary Fiber 4g	14%
Total Sugars 6g	
Includes 0g Added Sugars	0%
Protein 15g	
Vitamin D 0mcg	0%
Calcium 320mg	25%
Iron 1.6mg	8%
Potassium 510mg	10%

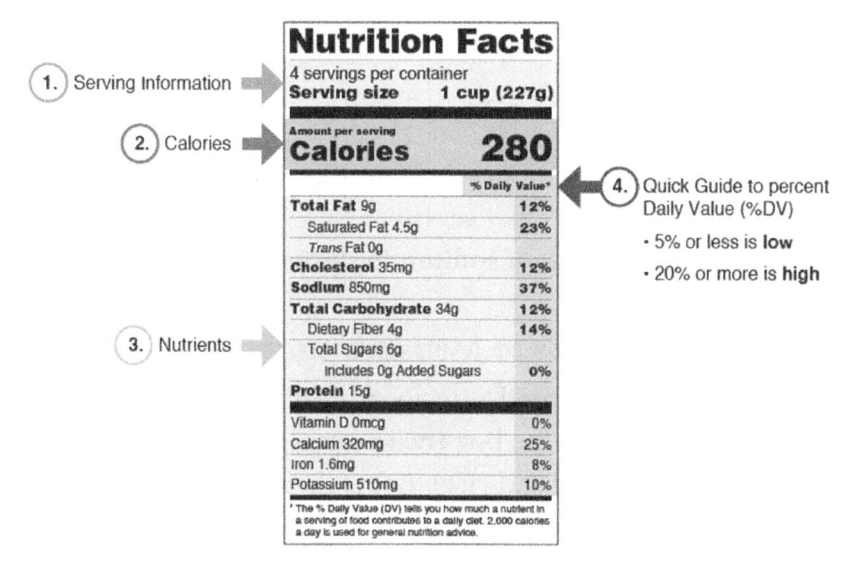

* The % Daily Value (DV) tells you how much a nutrient in a serving of food contributes to a daily diet. 2,000 calories a day is used for general nutrition advice.

Figure 3. FDA Nutrition Facts Label Frozen Lasagna Example[35]

Here are more examples:
- ☑ The milligrams (mg) of sodium in *one* serving is 850 mg
- ☑ The milligrams (mg) of sodium in *two* servings = 850 mg × 2 servings = 1,700 mg
- ☑ The grams (g) of fiber in *three* servings of the product = 4 grams × 3 servings = 12 g
- ☑ The grams (g) of carbohydrates in *one* serving of the product = 34 g
- ☑ And so on

Servings Per Container

The nutrition facts label has a line above the serving size that contains the "servings per container." Take a moment to identify the servings per container in Figure 3. Did you see that it contains four servings per container? Knowing this number allows us to calculate the nutrient content of the entire package.

To find the number of a particular nutrient in the entire package, multiply the servings per container (four in this case) by the grams/milligrams per serving of that nutrient. For example, let's use sodium again:

**4 servings per container x 850 milligrams of sodium per serving =
3,400 milligrams of sodium in the entire package**

Use Measuring Cups to Measure Servings

Sometimes, we eat food directly from the bag (hello chips), pour our servings from the box (hello cereal), or just scoop them on the plate (hello pasta and rice), not realizing how much we are eating. This leads to many of us eating more calories than we need. Next time, use a measuring cup to measure out a serving to get a more accurate account of how much of each nutrient you are taking in. This is not calorie counting; instead, consider this nutrient awareness.

A common serving size for cereal is two-thirds (2/3) cup. If you are not good with adding fractions in your head, like me, you can use a calculator to calculate more than one serving.

Serving Size Practice

Nutrition Facts
4 servings per container
Serving size 1 1/2 cup (208g)

Amount Per Serving
Calories 240

	% Daily Value*
Total Fat 4g	**5%**
Saturated Fat 1.5g	**8%**
Trans Fat 0g	
Cholesterol 5mg	**2%**
Sodium 430mg	**19%**
Total Carbohydrate 46g	**17%**
Dietary Fiber 7g	**25%**
Total Sugars 4g	
Includes 2g Added Sugars	**4%**
Protein 11g	
Vitamin D 2mcg	10%
Calcium 260mg	20%
Iron 6mg	35%
Potassium 240mg	6%

* The % Daily Value (DV) tells you how much a nutrient in a serving of food contributes to a daily diet. 2,000 calories a day is used for general nutrition advice.

Figure 4. FDA Nutrition Facts Label Example [36]

1. How many grams of total sugars are in *one serving* of the food item in Figure 4? _____
2. How many grams of total sugars are in *the entire package*? _____
3. How many grams of saturated fat are in *the entire package*? _____
4. How many milligrams of iron are in *two servings* of this food item? _____
5. How many cups are in *two servings* of this food item? _____

See answers in the endnotes.[37]

Nutrient Quantities

The nutrition facts labels include the quantities of several nutrients in grams or milligrams. These nutrients fall into two categories: macronutrients and micronutrients.

The Macronutrients

These are the nutrients you can see with the naked eye and are measured in grams (See more on macronutrients in chapters 14-16.). Cholesterol is the only macronutrient measured in milligrams. The macronutrients on the label include:
- Carbohydrates
  - Sugar
  - Added sugars
  - Fiber
- Protein
- Fats
  - Total fats
  - Saturated fats
- Cholesterol

The Micronutrients

These are the nutrients you cannot see with the naked eye, and they are measured in milligrams or micrograms (See more on micronutrients in Chapter 17.). The micronutrients on the nutrition facts label include:
- Minerals
  - Sodium
  - Potassium
  - Calcium
  - Iron
- Vitamins
  - Vitamin D

Except for sodium, the FDA chose these particular micronutrients for the label because many people don't get enough of them in their diets.

- ☑ Take a moment to look at these nutrients in Figures 2, 3, and 4.
- ☑ Check out the "% daily value" for each micronutrient on the label (More on the % daily value in the pages to come.).
- ☑ If the "% daily value" is greater than 20%, this is considered a good source of that particular nutrient. If the "% daily value" is less than 5%, it is not considered a good nutrient source. You can use this information to determine if it is a healthy food. Remember to check the ingredients list first, though. Some foods may be high in potassium, vitamin D, iron, and calcium but may still have not-so-good-for-you ingredients.

> Macronutrients include fats, carbohydrates and proteins.
> Micronutrients include vitamins and minerals.

What Does "Total Carbohydrate" Mean?

Carbohydrates consist of sugars, starches, and fiber. Total carbohydrates on the nutrition facts label, therefore, are the total grams of carbohydrates from sugars, starches, and fiber present in that particular food item. In Figure 5, note that only sugars and fibers, not starches, are listed separately.

Total Carbohydrate 46g	**17%**
Dietary Fiber 7g	**25%**
Total Sugars 4g	
Includes 2g Added Sugars	**4%**
Sugar Alcohol 0g	

Figure 5. FDA's Total Carbohydrates on Nutrition Facts Label Example

Recommendations for diabetes are beyond the scope of this book, but I feel the need to mention that if you have been diagnosed with diabetes or pre-diabetes, you will want to pay attention to total carbohydrates, not just sugar.

What Is the Difference Between Total Sugars and Added Sugars?

Let's start with added sugars.

Added Sugars

Some foods, like milk, dairy, and fruit, have natural sugars. It's the way nature made them. Added sugars are sugars extracted from plants that are then put into foods. Foods and drinks like chocolate milk, flavored yogurts, sweetened applesauce, and fruit cups with syrup have added sugars in addition to their natural sugars.

Total sugars
=
the total grams of natural sugars
+
added sugars

These extracted sugars are also added to foods that don't have any natural sugars, as is the case with things like cookies and soda. I do not recommend eliminating natural sugars. However, I do recommend reducing added sugars altogether. Pay attention to this "added sugars" number. Make sure it is a very low number (ideally, zero grams).

Total Sugars

Total sugars are the natural sugars plus added sugars. If the food item does not have any natural sugars, the total sugars will equal the added sugar amount.

The food item in Figure 6 has 2 grams of natural sugar because:

4 grams of total sugar-2 grams of added sugar
= 2 grams of natural sugar

```
Total Sugars 4g
Includes 2g Added Sugars         4%
```

Figure 6. FDA's Sugars on Nutrition Facts Label Example

The addition of added sugars to the nutrition facts label was a powerful development. Before this development, there was no way to determine how much added sugar was in a particular item.

What About Artificial Sweeteners and Sugar Alternatives?

Artificial sweeteners are created in a lab to add sweetness to our foods and drinks instead of added sugars. You cannot determine if an item has artificial sweeteners or sugar alternatives by looking at the sugar section on the nutrition facts label. If the nutrition facts label says "0 g" total sugar, the item can still have artificial sweeteners/sugar alternatives. Instead of the label, you have to look at the ingredients list.

To determine if your food item contains artificial sweeteners, look out for the common artificial sweetener names below on the ingredients list:

- Aspartame (NutraSweet, Equal)
- Acesulfame Potassium (Ace-K)
- Sucralose (Splenda)
- Neotame
- Advantame
- Saccharin (Sweet & Low)

"No Sugar Added" does not mean there are no artificial sweeteners.

Since I don't want to overwhelm you with all the names for artificial sweeteners, I will have you recall the reason why the "put it back on the shelf if you don't recognize the name on the ingredients list"

rule is so helpful. I do not recommend the consumption of artificial sweeteners for several reasons:
- ☑ Some people consume them for weight loss because they do not have any calories. However, there is no evidence to suggest that they aid in weight loss over the long term.[38]
- ☑ Others consume them for blood sugar control. However, evidence suggests they cause a worsened ability to control blood sugar.[39]
- ☑ Consumption may increase the risk for cancer, cardiovascular disease, and other ill-health effects.[40]

Sugar Alcohols

Sugar alcohols are chemically altered sugars and are not considered to be added sugars (see Figure 7). Unlike artificial sweeteners, they have calories but less calories than sugar. You may or may not find them on the nutrition facts label.

Total Carbohydrate 46g	**17%**
Dietary Fiber 7g	**25%**
Total Sugars 4g	
Includes 2g Added Sugars	**4%**
Sugar Alcohol 0g	

Figure 7. FDA's Sugar Alcohol on Nutrition Facts Label Example[41]

To determine if the food item contains sugar alcohols, look at the ingredients list, as it may not be listed on the label. They typically have the letters -ol at the end. Here are some names of commonly used sugar alcohols:
- Isomalt
- Lactitol

- Maltitol
- Mannitol
- Sorbitol
- Xylitol

An ingredient that ends in "-ol" is a sign that it is most likely a sugar alcohol.

I recommend staying away from sugar alcohols as well. They can cause bloating, diarrhea, abdominal pain, and gas, and they are associated with an increased risk of heart attacks and stroke.[42] Recall the "if you don't recognize it" rule to help you avoid sugar alcohol.

What About Alternatives Like Stevia and Agave?

Stevia and agave are natural sweeteners extracted from plants. While they seem to be healthy alternatives to sugar, remember that sugar is also a natural sweetener extracted from plants. Also, remember that the food industry is great at convincing us that foods are healthy even though there is no evidence to suggest that their claims are true. If you decide to use them, use them in moderation like you would sugar. Or don't use them at all.

Look at the ingredients list to determine if a food has stevia or agave.

Percent Daily Values (%DV)

Do you know what the % Daily Value means? You know the number with the percentage sign on the far right of the nutrition facts label (see Figure 8 below)?

	% Daily Value*
Total Fat 4g	**5%**
Saturated Fat 1.5g	**8%**
Trans Fat 0g	

Figure 8. FDA's % Daily Value Nutrition Facts Label Example

We need a certain amount of different types of nutrients to obtain optimal health. The % Daily Value is the percentage of those needs that *one serving* of a food item provides. Since we all have different needs, and they can only practically print one number per serving, the FDA uses a 2,000-calorie diet as the base to determine that percentage. This means that if your daily needs are 1,500 calories, you would need to adjust the percentage. However, the number is useful to give us a general idea.

Figure 9 is the chart that you will find on most packages to explain what the % percent daily value is based on. It also provides recommended amounts of different nutrients for individuals on a 2,000 and 2,500-calorie diet.

* Percent Daily Values are based on a 2,000 calorie diet. Your Daily Values may be higher or lower depending on your calorie needs.			
	Calories:	**2,000**	**2,500**
Total Fat	Less than	65g	80g
Sat Fat	Less than	20g	25g
Cholesterol	Less than	300mg	300mg
Sodium	Less than	2,400mg	2,400mg
Total Carbohydrate		300g	375g
Dietary Fiber		25g	30g

Figure 9. Percent Daily Value Chart found on Packaged Foods

Let's apply this practically using Figures 9 and 10:
- ☑ Per Figure 9, less than 20 grams of saturated fat per day is recommended for a person on a 2,000-calorie diet.
- ☑ The food item in Figure 10 below has 1.5 grams of saturated fat. If we do a little math to find the percent daily value, we get:

- 1.5 grams of saturated fat per serving divided by 20 recommended grams = 0.075
  - 0.075 * 100 = 7.5% rounded up to 8%
- ☑ This is where the 8% comes from, and it represents one serving.
- ☑ If you eat two servings, you will have eaten 16% (or 3 grams).
- ☑ If you eat the entire package, you will have eaten 32% (or 6 grams) of the recommended amount for the day because there are 4 servings in this container (Don't forget about the servings per container.).

Nutrition Facts

4 servings per container
Serving size 1 1/2 cup (208g)

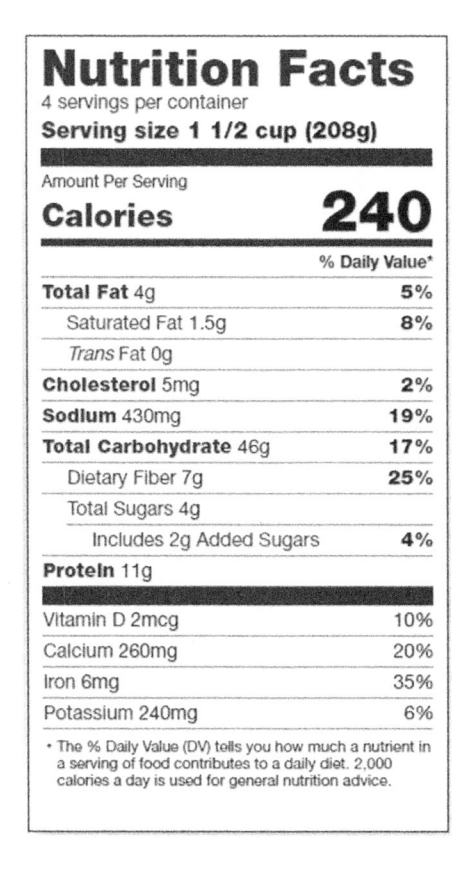

Amount Per Serving
Calories   **240**

	% Daily Value*
Total Fat 4g	5%
Saturated Fat 1.5g	8%
Trans Fat 0g	
Cholesterol 5mg	2%
Sodium 430mg	19%
Total Carbohydrate 46g	17%
Dietary Fiber 7g	25%
Total Sugars 4g	
Includes 2g Added Sugars	4%
Protein 11g	
Vitamin D 2mcg	10%
Calcium 260mg	20%
Iron 6mg	35%
Potassium 240mg	6%

* The % Daily Value (DV) tells you how much a nutrient in a serving of food contributes to a daily diet. 2,000 calories a day is used for general nutrition advice.

Figure 10. FDA Nutrition Facts Label Example

Percent Daily Value (% DV) Quiz Time. Use Figure 10 above to answer the questions.
1. What % of the recommended sodium for the day is in *one* serving of this product? _____
2. What % of the recommended sodium for the day is in *three* servings of this product? _____
3. What % of the recommended fiber for the day is in *two* servings of this product? _____
4. What % of the recommended potassium for the day is in *one* serving of this product? _____

See the answers are in the endnotes[43]

Apply Your Knowledge

Based on what you know about the product in Figure 10 so far, without knowing what the food item is, do you think that this is a healthy food?

Here are the things I would consider:

The Good
- ☑ The product has a good amount of calcium, iron, protein, and fiber.
- ☑ It has a moderate amount of vitamin D.
- ☑ The product is also low in sugar, cholesterol, and saturated fat and is not too bad on calories.

The Not so Good
- ☑ The product has a hefty amount of sodium.

So far, the good significantly outweighs the not-so-good for me. But remember, if sodium is a big concern for you, then you should weigh it more heavily. Setting rules can be helpful. Let's say I have a rule of no more than 300 mg of sodium per serving. That might be all I need to look at to rule it out as an option for me.

This is somewhat of a trick question, though. You cannot determine whether this is a healthy food without the ingredients list. Here is a recap of steps you can take:
1. Evaluate the ingredients list to ensure they are all whole foods you recognize as healthy.
2. Go to the nutrition facts label, and weigh the good, bad, and ugly, as we did above.
3. Then make your choice.

If the ingredients are foods that I recognize as healthy, I would consider this a healthy choice. If you are just trying to find something not so bad and not necessarily healthy, use these general rules:
1. Choose the one with fewer unrecognizable ingredients.
2. Then choose the one with fewer saturated fat, cholesterol, sodium, and total sugars.
3. Choose the one with more fiber and protein.
4. Finally, choose the one with a higher percentage of calcium, vitamin D, iron, or potassium (20% or more is considered a good source).

Again, it may not be "healthy" per our definition, but it will most likely be a healthier choice.

The More You Use It

Reading the nutrition facts label can be overwhelming initially, but the more you do it, the easier it gets. And don't worry if you shop online; the nutrition facts label is there too. You, therefore, have this information at your fingertips, even if you are not in the store.

Now let's take a closer look at the nutrients listed on the label. Starting with carbohydrates.

CHAPTER 14

CARBOHYDRATES

From chapters 12 and 13, we know that there are three macronutrients that the body needs to function optimally: Carbohydrates, fats, and proteins. But which version of these macronutrients should we consume for optimal health? This and the following two chapters will clarify many of your questions. Let's start with carbohydrates or carbs.

What Are Carbohydrates?

Carbohydrates are a series of carbon and hydrogen atoms bound together to create sugar, starches (which turn into sugar after eating), and fiber. The main goal of that sugar is to provide the body with energy). The body then uses that energy to function.

Fiber regulates how we use sugar, keeps the colon clean, lowers cholesterol, fills us up, and provides a breeding ground for good bacteria in the gut. Having a healthy gut is one of the most powerful things you can do for your health. Making fiber one of the most powerful nutrients that we can consume for our health.

> The three main carbohydrates are:
> Sugars
> Starches and
> Fiber

Some foods have one or a combination of these three groups of carbohydrates. For example, beans have starch, fiber, and some sugar, while white pasta is mostly starch. Sugars, starches, and fiber fall into one of two categories: simple and complex carbs. Here's the difference between the two:

Simple Carbohydrates are also known as sugars and are the most basic unit of a carbohydrate. The main sugars that we eat are glucose, galactose, and fructose, and almost every other carbohydrate is built from a combination of these three. Imagine a chain with multiple links. Simple carbohydrates (glucose, galactose, and fructose) are like the individual links in the chain.

When food or drink is composed mostly of simple carbohydrates/sugar (like soda or candy), the body digests the food quickly and almost immediately causes an increase in blood sugar, which is often called a blood sugar spike. You are less likely to experience a spike with complex carbohydrates.

Complex Carbohydrates are your starches and fibers. If simple carbohydrates/sugars are the individual links in the chain, starches and fibers are the chains. Some of these chains have branches and can get all kinds of complicated in how they are structured. Because they are more complicated, they don't digest as quickly as simple sugars.

Fiber is the most complex and does not break down into sugar like starches do. For all intents and purposes, fiber does not have calories, so we don't get much energy from fiber. However, its role is equally important as it cleanses the colon, creates healthy gut bacteria, and slows digestion.

Let's look at fruit. Fruit combines a simple carb (sugar) with a complex carb (fiber). Therefore, when we eat fruit, our blood sugar doesn't spike as drastically as it does when we drink orange juice. That is because the fiber in fruit slows down the digestion of the sugar. Orange juice has nothing to slow down the digestion of sugar, which is why it spikes sugar levels in the blood almost immediately.

Where Are Carbohydrates Found?

Sugars (simple carbs) are found in fruit, milk, and sweeteners like sugar, honey, agave, and syrups. Sweeteners like stevia are not sugar, even though they are sweet.

Starches (the complex carbs) are found in bread, pasta, rice, cereals, grains (like oats, wheat, and quinoa), beans, lentils, corn, peas, potatoes, plantains, and winter squashes.

> Simple Carbohydrates = Sugars
>
> Complex Carbohydrates = Starches and Fiber

Fiber is found in fruits, vegetables, 100% whole grains, beans, nuts, and seeds. Recall that fiber passes through the body mainly undigested and, therefore, for all intents and purposes, does not have calories.

— TABLE 14.1 —
TYPES OF CARBOHYDRATES IN COMMON FOODS AND DRINKS

FOODS WITH SUGAR (SIMPLE CARBS)	FOODS WITH STARCH (COMPLEX CARBS)	FOODS WITH FIBER (COMPLEX CARBS)
Fruit Milk Sweeteners Sweets Sweetened beverages	Beans Lentils Bread Pasta Rice Other grains (like oats) Starchy vegetables (like corn, peas, and potatoes)	Fruit Beans Lentils Vegetables Nuts Seeds Bread (100% whole only) Pasta (100% whole only) Rice (Brown only) Other grains (100% whole only)

Simple versus complex is one way to classify carbohydrates in general. These classifications don't necessarily tell us if the food is healthy or not. The refined or whole classifications can give us some insights into how healthy a carbohydrate may be. You may have heard the term whole grain. You might consider the opposite of a whole grain a refined grain. Let's get into it.

Whole Grains vs. Refined Grains

Grains are different types of edible grasses like wheat, barley, rye, rice, oats, and quinoa. As mentioned in the previous section, grains contain complex carbs (starches and fibers). Bread, pasta, and cereals are considered grains because they are made primarily from grains, especially wheat. Grains are either whole or refined.

Whole grains have not been changed much from their original form and have most of their nutrients intact. Not only do they contain starches and fiber (which we now know are complex carbohydrates), but they also have healthy fats, protein, vitamins, and minerals. The fiber, protein, and healthy fats in whole grains help to stabilize blood sugar and are helpful for preventing and managing diabetes. They also fill us up faster, so we are less likely to eat as much. This makes it helpful for weight management and aging compared to refined grains.

> When choosing whole grains, make sure the package says "100% whole" for optimal nutrition.

Refined grains are whole grains that have been stripped of many of their nutrients. Food manufacturers remove these nutrients so that the product can last longer on store shelves. Refined grains are sometimes called white grains (e.g., white bread, white pasta, and white rice).

After removing the nutrients, they "enrich" the product by replacing some of the vitamins they removed. They do not replace the fiber, healthy fats, protein, minerals, and many of the vitamins that they removed. The final product is mostly starch and a few vitamins.

Stripping whole grains of fiber, fat, and protein to create refined grains means that there is nothing to slow down the digestion of the starch. This also means that refined grains like white bread, rice, and pasta can make blood sugar levels go up almost as fast as sugar itself. Removing these nutrients is also why they are not as filling as whole grains, making us more likely to eat more. We encourage 100% whole grains in place of refined grains because refined grains are thought to be a major contributor to the development of diabetes and obesity.

If whole grains are healthier than refined grains, can you eat all the whole grains you want? No. Certain grains (including wheat, barley, and rye) contain gluten. Many have gluten sensitivities and do not even know it (more on gluten later). 100% whole grains also have a significant number of calories from carbohydrates that can also lead to weight gain. Let's look at the quantity of carbohydrates that may promote optimal health.

> The term "enriched" on the ingredients label on a package means that the manufacturer replaced *some* of the vitamins they removed.

How Many Grams of Carbohydrates Do We Need?

The Recommended Dietary Allowance (RDA) can help us answer this question. According to the National Institutes of Health (NIH), "An RDA is the average daily dietary intake level sufficient to meet the nutrient requirements of nearly all (97–98 percent) healthy individuals in a group".[44] A "group" is categorized by age, gender, pregnancy status, and lactation status. The RDA for carbohydrates for males and females who are not pregnant or lactating is **130 grams** of carbohydrates a day (or 520 calories from carbohydrates).

This is a significant difference from what is on the nutrition facts label, which is more akin to the typical American dietary intake.

> The carbohydrate Recommended Dietary Allowance (RDA) for males and females who are not pregnant, or lactating is **130 grams** of carbohydrates a day—a significant difference from what is used by the USDA on the nutrition facts label.

What the USDA Says About the Matter

The USDA recommends that 45%-65% of our total daily calories come from carbohydrates. Remember BMR from Chapter 12? If your BMR is 1,500 calories a day, 45%-65% of 1,500 works out to 675–975 calories from carbohydrates which is 167-245 grams of carbohydrates.

The nutrition facts label is based on a 2,000-calorie diet and they use 300 grams of carbohydrates as the basis for the percent daily value (%DV). So, if a food product has 45 grams of carbohydrates per serving, the %DV *on the label* will be 15% (45 grams is 15% of 300 grams). That math is already done for you on the label.

Comparing the Nutrition Facts Label to the RDA

See Table 14.1 to compare the %DV on the nutrition facts label versus what the %DV would be if we used the RDA of 130 grams to determine the %DV.

— TABLE 14.1 —
PERCENT DAILY VALUE (%DV) COMPARISON FOR COMMONLY EATEN CARBOHYDRATES

FOOD	SERVING SIZE	APPROXIMATE GRAMS OF CARBOHYDRATES PER SERVING	%DV PER THE NUTRITION FACTS LABEL (300 GRAMS/DAY TOTAL)	%DV PER THE RDA (130 GRAMS/DAY TOTAL)
Rice	1 cup	45	15%	35%
Beans	1 cup	45	15%	35%
Pasta	1 cup	35	12%	27%
Bread	2 slices	30	10%	23%
White Potato	1 large	25	8%	19%
Handheld fruit	1 medium	25	8%	19%
Berries	1 cup	20	7%	15%
Milk	1 cup	12	4%	9%
Non-Starchy Veggies* (all you can eat)	-	-	0%	0%
Total		237	80%	184%

*Non-starchy veggies include things like lettuce, kale, collard and other greens, brussels sprouts, and more. They are often called "free carbs" because their carb content is negligible after we account for their fiber. More information on net carbs to come.

If we ate the 237 grams of carbohydrates, represented in Table 14.1, in one day, we would eat 184% of what our body needs for the day, per the RDA (or 84% more than what we need). If we use the label numbers, we would think we are eating 80%, (or 20% less than what we need.).

Why mention this? To clarify the information on the label. The nutrition facts label is useful for the approximate amounts of calories and other nutrients that are in specific products. However, the % DV can be misleading for a large percentage of the healthy American population. So, when you see the %DV for carbohydrates, know that your needs may differ from someone who needs 300 grams of carbohydrates a day. In fact, it may be closer to someone who needs 130 grams a day.

Fruits and Vegetables Have Less Carbohydrates and More Fiber than Grains

You might look at Table 14.1 and say, but hey, beans have a lot of carbs. And I would say, true, but beans also have a lot of carbohydrates from fiber. I can eat larger portions of veggies and beans without worrying about all the calories that come with other foods that don't have as much fiber.

Many of us will place two cups of rice or pasta on our plate without giving it a second thought, not realizing that this adds up to about 60%-70% of what our body requires for the day. To help with this, use measuring cups and pay attention to serving sizes. It helps keep your carbohydrate intake in check and saves money!

> Non-starchy vegetables like lettuce and greens are considered "free carbs" in some circles because their fiber content is so high, and starch/sugar content is so low.

How Many Grams of Carbohydrates Are You Eating?

Before continuing with this section, I want to reiterate that I don't provide this information because I want you to obsess about counting calories or grams of carbs, fat, and protein. Instead, it is to create awareness of what we need compared to what we eat. Once we get a sense of what our body can handle, it will help us make different choices. Choices like asking the server in the burrito bowl line to give us one scoop of rice instead of two large scoops or ordering the child-sized ice cream instead of the large.

> Searching for the number of carbohydrates in a serving size of a particular food is a helpful reference, but it can become overwhelming. The best way to ensure you are not giving your body more than it can handle is by prioritizing whole unprocessed foods, especially those with fiber, and watching portion sizes. Otherwise, use those nutrition facts labels!

We have a general sense of the amount of carbohydrates most people need for the day: about 130 grams (some require less, some require more). Now, let's look at how much we are actually eating.

Again, you can find the approximate amount of carbohydrates (sugars, starches, and fibers) in a particular product by:

- ☑ Reading the nutrition facts label.
- ☑ Using the USDA FoodData Central website: https://fdc.nal.usda.gov/.
- ☑ Using a calorie counting app.

For cooked grains and beans, the servings are listed as cooked, dried, or by a fraction of the package (e.g., 1/8 of a box). Table 14.2 is a guide translating what that means.

— TABLE 14.2 —
SERVING SIZES OF CERTAIN COOKED VERSUS DRIED CARBOHYDRATES

	CARBOHYDRATES PER SERVING – DRIED VS. COOKED			
FOOD	TYPICAL SERVING SIZE ON NUTRITION FACTS LABEL	TRANSLATES TO ABOUT…	GRAMS OF CARBOHYDRATES PER SERVING	%DV PER THE RDA *(130 GRAMS/ DAY TOTAL)*
Rice	"¼ cup dry"	¾ cup cooked	35	27%
Beans	"¼ cup dry"	¾ cup cooked	35	27%
Pasta	"2 ounces dry"	½ - 1 cup cooked *(depending on the type of pasta)*	20-40	15%-31%
Oatmeal	"½ cup dry"	1 cup cooked	30	23%
Quinoa	"¼ cup dry"	¾ cup cooked	31	24%
Split Peas	"¼ cup dry"	½ cup cooked	22	17%

What About Net Carbohydrates (Net Carbs)

Net carbs are the carbohydrates that we get calories from. Recall:

- ☑ We know that starches, sugar, and fiber are carbohydrates.
- ☑ Starches and sugars are carbohydrates that contain calories (about 4 calories per gram).
- ☑ However, fiber contains no calories for all intents and purposes as it goes mostly undigested.
- ☑ Since fiber does not have calories, we subtract the number of grams of fiber from the total number of carbohydrates to get the approximate number of calories from carbs. Those are your net carbs.

Calculating Net Carbs Example
If total carbs = 40 grams
and fiber = 5 grams
then net carbs = 40 grams – 5 grams
= 35 grams

Tables 14.3 and 14.4 provide the approximate number of grams of total and net carbs there are in the most common carbohydrate-rich foods from least to most net carbs.

— TABLE 14.3 —
TOTAL AND NET CARBOHYDRATES IN COMMON STARCHY FOODS

COMPLEX CARBOHYDRATES (I.E. FOOD RICH IN STARCH OR FIBER)	SERVING SIZE	GRAMS OF CARBS PER SERVING	NET CARBS PER SERVING
Non-starchy veggies (celery, carrots, greens, etc.)	1 cup raw	1-10 grams	1-5 grams
Winter squash (e.g., butternut)	1 cup cooked	15 grams	13 grams
Sweet peas	1 cup cooked	24 grams	17 grams
Cream of wheat	1 cup cooked	20 grams	20 grams
Corn	1 cup cooked	30 grams	25 grams
Lentils	1 cup cooked	40 grams	25 grams
Oatmeal	1 cup cooked	30 grams	25 grams
Sweet potatoes (medium potato)	1 cup cooked	30 grams	25 grams
White potatoes (medium potato)	1 cup cooked	30 grams	25 grams
Whole wheat/grain bread	2 slices	30 grams	26 grams
Beans	1 cup cooked	45 grams	30 grams
Potato/plantain chips	15 chips	30 grams	30 grams
White bread	2 slices	30 grams	30 grams
Sweetened cereals	1 cup	35 grams	35 grams
Quinoa	1 cup cooked	40 grams	35 grams
Whole wheat/grain cereals	1 cup	45 grams	35 grams
Brown rice	1 cup cooked	45 grams	40 grams
Whole wheat/grain pasta	1 cup cooked	45 grams	40 grams
White pasta	1 cup cooked	45 grams	43 grams
Plantains	1 medium	50 grams	45 grams
White rice	1 cup cooked	45 grams	45 grams
Yuca (cassava)	1 cup cooked	50 grams	48 grams

*To calculate fiber per serving, subtract grams of carbs per serving from net carbs.

— TABLE 14.4 —
TOTAL AND NET CARBOHYDRATES IN POPULAR NON-STARCHY FOODS

SIMPLE CARBOHYDRATES (I.E. FOOD WITH SUGARS)	SERVING SIZE	GRAMS OF CARBS PER SERVING	NET CARBS PER SERVING
Almond Milk (Unsweetened)	1 cup	3 grams	3 grams
Milk	1 cup	12 grams	12 grams
Sugar (White)	1 tablespoon	12 grams	12 grams
Maple syrup	1 tablespoon	13 grams	13 grams
Molasses	1 tablespoon	13 grams	13 grams
Agave	1 tablespoon	15 grams	15 grams
Fruit (apple, orange, pear, etc.)	1 small	20 grams	15 grams
Fruit (berries)	1 cup	20 grams	16 grams
Raw honey	1 tablespoon	17 grams	17 grams
Ice Cream (Vanilla)	1 cup	35 grams	35 grams
Soda/Pop	1 cup	30 grams	30 grams

*To calculate calories, multiply the net carbs by 4 (there are 4 calories in every gram of net carbohydrates).

Exercise: How Many Carbohydrates?

1. Use tables 14.3 and 14.4 and take a moment to record the carbohydrates you eat in a typical day. List the food item and grams of net carbs below or on a separate sheet of paper. Then add them together to get the total. If a food you eat is not listed, like lasagna, break it down and make an estimate. Lasagna has carbs from the pasta and a little from the ricotta cheese. If you think there is about one cup of pasta in that lasagna, use 45 grams of carbs as your number. It's the same with pizza. If you eat one large slice or two small slices of pizza, use 2 slices of bread or 30 grams of carbs.

    Remember to record portion sizes—if you eat more or less than one cup of mashed potatoes, account for that. Two cups of mashed potatoes would be 60 grams of carbohydrates, one-half cup would be 15 grams, and so on. It does not need to be a perfect account, just a rough estimate to help you see where you are.

E.g. Food Item <u>4 slices of white bread</u>, grams of Net Carbs <u> 60 </u>

Food Item _____, grams of Net Carbs _____

Food Item _____, grams of Net Carbs _____

Food Item _____, grams of Net Carbs _____

Food Item _____, grams of Net Carbs _____

Food Item _____, grams of Net Carbs _____

Food Item _____, grams of Net Carbs _____

Food Item _____, grams of Net Carbs _____

Food Item _____, grams of Net Carbs _____

Food Item _____, grams of Net Carbs _____

Food Item _____, grams of Net Carbs _____

Food Item _____, grams of Net Carbs _____

Food Item _____, grams of Net Carbs _____

Food Item _____, grams of Net Carbs _____

Food Item _____, grams of Net Carbs _____

Food Item _____, grams of Net Carbs _____

Food Item _____, grams of Net Carbs _____

Food Item _____, grams of Net Carbs _____

Food Item _____, grams of Net Carbs _____

Food Item _____, grams of Net Carbs _____

Food Item _____, grams of Net Carbs _____

TOTAL _____

2. Compare your total to 130 grams.
3. If your number is between 100 and 200 grams, you are doing well!
4. If your number exceeds 250 grams, consider whether that is appropriate for your activity levels, height, and weight (use BMR as a guide). If it is not, consider replacing some higher-carb options with lower-carb options (My rice cakes instead of bagels, for example.). And remember, you can start with one change at a time.
5. If your number is below 100 grams, make sure it is because you are choosing healthy carbs with protein and fiber, like non-starchy vegetables, beans, and lentils. Otherwise, ensure you are getting enough to meet your nutrient needs (again, use your BMR as a guide).

Remember, the purpose of this activity is not to stress you out about numbers but instead to create awareness of whether we are overworking our bodies by eating too many (or too few) carbohydrates.

Do You Ever Need to "Load up" on the Carbohydrates

Loading up on carbohydrates is not necessary unless you do high-intensity physical activity for hours at a time. You want to "load up" in these instances because carbohydrates offer a quick supply of energy that you can access more easily than the energy we get from fat.

When running a marathon, for example, you want to ensure you have enough energy to make it through the race. Carb loading allows for this. At any other time, carb loading is not necessary.

Is "Good" vs. "Bad" Carbohydrates a Thing?

We know that different foods have different types of carbohydrates (sugars, starches, and fiber). We also understand how natural, unprocessed foods can be altered to the point where a lot, if not most, of the nutrition is removed and that these are called processed foods. Some foods are slightly processed (like oats), and other foods are ultra-processed (like cookies and sugar-sweet cereals). White flour used to make breads and baked goods is an ultra-processed form of wheat.

So, are there "good" and "bad carbs? YES. Natural (unprocessed) carbohydrates like those found in whole fruit and beans that cause no harm to most can be considered good carbohydrates. Ultra-processed foods like refined (white) sugar and flour (or foods that contain these foods) can cause harm and I would consider them to be "bad."

Again, there is some debate among health professionals as to whether using "good" vs. "bad" is the best way to classify food. And again, I have no hesitation in using those terms. It's simple if you are defining good versus bad based on its impact on health. But instead of looking at them as "good" vs "bad," let's just consider them "healthy" and "unhealthy" carbohydrates to match our definition of healthy.[45]

DO LOAD UP ON FIBER

The recommendation (or Dietary Reference Intake) for total fiber is 26 grams for adult females and 38 grams for adult males.

- ☑ One cup of beans or lentils has 8-16 grams of fiber.
- ☑ An apple or pear has about 4-5 grams.
- ☑ Carrots, beets, broccoli, kale, sweet potatoes, and other vegetables contain about 2-4 grams of fiber per cup.
- ☑ Oats and quinoa, about 4 grams per cup.
- ☑ Nuts and seeds about 2 grams per ¼ cup.

Animal products do not contain fiber, but fiber starts to add up quickly when we focus on plant-based foods. This is one of many reasons why eating mostly plants, including the three vegetables and two fruits per day recommendation, is important for optimal health.

Calculate the grams of fiber you eat in a day using Tables 14.3 and 14.4. Are you close to the recommendation?

Eating a little bit of, say, refined (white) sugar probably won't cause any harm. As long as it is in moderation, it shouldn't be a problem then, right? I still classify it as "unhealthy." Why? Because some foods contribute to the body functioning at maximum capacity (and therefore, promote optimal health). Other foods put demands on the body that reduce the body's capacity to function optimally.

> A "healthy food" for the purposes of this book, is a food that promotes optimal health while doing no harm.

When functioning optimally, the body is poised to fight the ill effects of pollution, infections, viruses, and other attacks. It is also designed to rejuvenate itself every minute of every day, and it does an amazing job when given what it needs. But when the body does what it does naturally, **and** then it has to work harder or figure out what to do with a substance it wasn't designed to process naturally, that extra stress can be harmful.

Think about how you feel when you've been hired to do a specific job, and then your employer piles on a bunch of responsibilities that have nothing to do with the original job you were hired for. You are expected to do the original job and all the extra responsibilities. When you prove you are capable, the employer might want to stretch you a bit more and assign you tasks in an area you were not trained in. Not only do you have to complete the extra task, but you have to teach yourself how to do it. You may (or may not) enjoy the extra work and the challenge of learning a new skill all your own.

As you continue to show your competence in handling everything skillfully, your employer may keep piling on the responsibilities. You work harder and harder, keeping up with the demands, and he/she keeps piling it on. Perhaps you've even had that boss who will give you all the extra responsibilities but not the extra resources, no raise, and no promotion. Eventually, you burn out.

Our body's organs, reactions, and systems are the same way, and we act either as the fair boss or the boss who piles it on. This piling on can lead to organ failure and disease.

> There are good/healthy and bad/unhealthy carbohydrates. It's ok to acknowledge that. What is not ok is feeling guilty and beating ourselves up when we eat the bad/unhealthy.

So yeah, there are good/healthy and bad/unhealthy carbohydrates. It's ok to acknowledge that. What is not okay is feeling guilty and beating ourselves up when we eat the bad/unhealthy. More on this in Chapter 19.

To help sort through the "healthy" and "unhealthy" carbohydrates, Tables 14.5 and 14.6 list foods with carbohydrates, their level of processing, and whether they have fiber. The healthiest options are unprocessed foods with fiber.

— TABLE 14.5 —
PROCESSING LEVEL OF FOODS HIGH IN SUGAR

SUGAR OR FOODS WITH SUGAR	UNPROCESSED	MINIMALLY PROCESSED	ULTRA PROCESSED	CONTAINS FIBER
Fruit	X			X
Raw honey	X			
Honey			X	
Real maple syrup		X		
Pancake syrup			X	
Molasses		X		
Milk		X		
Plant-based milk			X	
Agave			X	
Sugar (cane, brown) and high fructose corn syrup.			X	
Ice cream			X	
Sweets (candy, cookies, cakes, doughnuts, etc.)			X	
Sugary beverages (sweetened sodas, energy drinks, iced teas, lemonades, etc.)			X	

*For optimal health, choose unprocessed or minimally processed foods with fiber. Also note that stevia and artificial sweeteners are not carbohydrates, even though they are sweeteners.

— TABLE 14.6 —
PROCESSING LEVEL OF FOODS HIGH IN STARCH

FOODS WITH STARCHES	UNPROCESSED	MINIMALLY PROCESSED	ULTRA PROCESSED	CONTAIN FIBER
Oatmeal		X		X
Quinoa		X		X
Brown rice		X		X
Beans	X			X
Lentils	X			X
Corn	X			X
Sweet peas	X			X
White potatoes	X			X
Sweet potatoes or yams	X			X
Plantains	X			X
Yuca (cassava)	X			X
Winter squash (e.g., butternut)	X			X
100% Whole wheat/grain bread		X		X
100% Whole wheat/grain pasta		X		X
100% Whole wheat/grain cereals		X		X
White rice			X	
White bread			X	
White pasta			X	
Cream of Wheat			X	
Most sweetened cereals			X	Depends
Potato/plantain chips			X	

*For optimal health, choose unprocessed or minimally processed foods with fiber. Also, note that whole/multi-grains should be 100% whole—if they are not 100%, they have been stripped of their nutrients.

Cow's Milk vs. Plant-Based Milk

Milk is a nutritious carbohydrate (a simple sugar) that has protein and fat. But there are cons associated with drinking milk, leaving space for alternatives like soy, coconut, almond and oat milk. However, there are negatives associated with the alternatives too. What's a person to do?

The key for either is to be moderate with consumption (For me, that is no more than 3-4 servings a week.). If you decide not to drink either, that is ok too. You don't need animal or plant-based milk for optimal health. All the nutrients found in either can be obtained by eating other foods. Table 14.7 lists some of the pros and cons of each to help you decide which one is right for you if you do drink them.

— TABLE 14.7 —
PROS AND CONS OF COW'S MILK VS. PLANT-BASED MILK

	COW'S MILK	PLANT-BASED MILK
PROS	✓ Contains natural protein, calcium, B12, vitamins A and D, and other vitamins and minerals ✓ May build stronger bones and teeth and may prevent osteoporosis	✓ No animal cruelty ✓ No hormones or antibiotics ✓ Lower environmental impact (Although almond milk has a higher water footprint.)[46]
CONS	✓ Animal cruelty is a strong possibility. ✓ More carbon emissions and water waste, which are harmful to the planet[47] ✓ Often contains hormones and antibiotics ✓ Pasteurization destroys some nutrition ✓ Consumption is associated with an increased risk of asthma and allergies[48] ✓ Lactose intolerance is a common problem ✓ Having worked with thousands of people, several have resolved symptoms of different diseases by eliminating milk and dairy from their diets	✓ Little to no natural protein, calcium, or B12 (sometimes, it is added) ✓ Health impacts have not been extensively evaluated over the long term, and we are not sure if they are harmful to health yet (except for coconut milk, which has clear health benefits.) ✓ Usually costs more than dairy milk

Now that you are an expert at reading nutrition facts labels and using the ingredients lists, use them to choose the plant-based milk right for you. Since plant-based milks are ultra-processed, I would not rank one above the other (Except coconut milk. It is less processed and has proven health benefits. I recommend above the others.). As mentioned in Chapter 13, I caution against choosing the ones with ingredients that you don't recognize and paying attention to the nutrients. Some have fat and a lot more calories than others. Others don't have as many vitamins and minerals, so beware.

What to Do When Conflicting Views About Certain Carbohydrates Surface

In case I didn't hammer down the point enough, I want to emphasize that natural, unprocessed carbohydrates, naturally high in fiber, are the best sources of carbohydrates. Some individuals may have seemingly extreme views about foods that fall even into these categories. For example, some say to avoid bananas and grapes because they're too high in sugar/carbohydrates. Some say to stay away from carrots because of the carbohydrate content (which is very low by most standards). Some say to stay away from *all* whole grains, including oats. When you hear things like this, I encourage you to put things into perspective.

> **OTHER MILKS**
>
> **A2 milk** is cow's milk with a protein (A2) that allows certain individuals with milk protein allergies/intolerances to consume milk without side effects. There are no extra health benefits from drinking this milk.
>
> **Goat's milk** is believed to have some health benefits over cow's milk (i.e., it's easier to digest and may not cause allergies). However, it is not essential for optimal health and is more expensive than cow's milk.
>
> **Raw milk** comes straight from the animal and is not pasteurized or altered. While there are significant benefits to drinking raw milk, selling it in most states is illegal because it may contain bacteria and cause illness.

> **Perspective 1:** What's the alternative for you? Would eating a cookie be better than eating that banana or those grapes? Would eating a potato chip be better than eating those carrots? Would

eating a sugary, sweet cereal be better than eating a bowl of oatmeal? If these claims concern you, by all means, reduce your intake, but always keep in mind the alternative for your budget and lifestyle.

Perspective 2: Do you have a specific health condition where you should avoid those foods? If yes, then avoid it. Otherwise, there are health benefits from natural whole foods. Even the ones higher on the carbohydrate/sugar content scale. The important thing is always moderation. If we eat four bananas, four cups of grapes, and two cups of oatmeal every day, that's a lot of sugar and carbohydrates, even if it is natural. That does not mean that the food is bad and that we should eliminate it from our diets. It just means we might want to chill on how much we eat. *Non-starchy* vegetables are the only foods I give the green light on eating with abandon as long as we eat various colors.

Perspective 3: How does your body respond to that particular food? If you don't feel good after eating it or have an allergy, then obviously avoid it. Or if you feel like eating that particular food causes you to gain or lose weight or counters some of your health goals, avoid it. Otherwise, it is fair game.

Stick to the basics, and don't allow extreme views to confuse you.

What About Gluten?

Gluten is a protein found in wheat, barley, and rye (sometimes oats if they are processed in a factory or grown where there is wheat, barley, or rye). It gives food that chewy sensation that we love so much. Most of the gluten we eat comes from wheat or products made from wheat or wheat flour (e.g., bread, pasta, cereals, pancakes, waffles, cookies, cakes, etc.). So even though gluten is a protein, it is embedded in a sea of carbohydrates.

Should You Avoid Gluten?

If you have a health condition that requires you to avoid gluten, like celiac disease, or if you have an allergy, obviously, you want to avoid gluten. Also, if you have a sensitivity to gluten, you also want to avoid gluten. Sensitivities are harder to detect than allergies because allergies come with an almost immediate reaction. Sensitivities may have less immediate reactions, making us less likely to connect our health issues to gluten intake.

My inflammatory eye flare-ups stopped when I significantly reduced my gluten intake. I went from eating gluten multiple times a day to eating it once a week or less. Pay attention to how much gluten you eat over a week. Reduce or eliminate gluten and see if it improves your health. See Table 14.8 for common sources of gluten. You might find that gluten is contributing to your stomach pain, flare-up, arthritic pain, nausea or whatever other symptom you may be experiencing.

If there are so many health conditions associated with gluten consumption, should we be eating it at all? At the very least, we could stand to reduce how much we eat. First, because the gluten we eat today is different from the gluten people ate years ago. It is more durable and more difficult for the body to process today, which may be why so many of us have allergies and sensitivities.

Second, because many of the ultra-processed foods that we eat contain gluten. The combination of sugar, flour, additives, etc., is a recipe for poor health, so it is not gluten alone causing so many problems, but a combination of factors.

Be aware of what foods contain gluten and consider reducing how much you eat (see Table 14.8). Set a goal for yourself, even if it's four instead of six servings of gluten a day. If you eat a breakfast sandwich, a slice of pizza, and a cookie for lunch, then chicken and pasta for dinner, you will have eaten 6-8 servings of grains with gluten. Something like swapping out a piece of fruit for a cookie could be a swap you could make that can make a difference.

Beware that gluten-free alternatives can be expensive and ultra-processed. That is where things like collard green wraps instead of bread, zoodles (noodles made with zucchini), or quinoa instead of pasta can come in handy.

Also, try to stick to the unprocessed versions of gluten. Barley, for example, is great for soups and as a side instead of pasta. It has gluten, but it's not processed. Table 14.8 has common processed sources of gluten to consider reducing if you are experiencing health problems.

— TABLE 14.8 —
POPULAR PROCESSED SOURCES OF GLUTEN

POPULAR SOURCES OF GLUTEN
Baked goods made with wheat (cookies, cakes, brownies, etc.)
Breaded fried foods
Crackers made with wheat flour
Cream of Wheat
Croutons and breadcrumbs
Flour made with wheat
Flour tortillas made with wheat
Cereals made with wheat
Rye (including rye bread)
Waffles/pancakes/French toast/biscuits made with wheat flour
White bread/bagels made with wheat flour
White pasta and noodles made with wheat
Whole wheat/grain bread
Whole wheat/grain cereals
Whole wheat/grain pasta

To determine if a product not listed here contains gluten, look for any ingredient on the ingredients list that includes the word "wheat" (enriched wheat flour, wheat protein, wheat bran, etc.), barley, or rye. You can also look for the words "gluten-free" to make sure a product does not contain gluten. Fruits, vegetables, beans, seeds, and nuts do not have gluten.

What Happens When You Eat Too Many Carbohydrates?

Remember, all carbohydrates (except fiber) are either sugar themselves or eventually break down into sugar in the blood. Three main things happen when there is too much sugar in the body:
1. It gets stored as fat.
2. It floats around in the blood.
3. It gets excreted into urine.

This combination of factors can lead to diseases like diabetes and heart disease.

Carbohydrates—The Takeaway

Carbohydrates come in many forms (simple vs complex, whole vs. refined, processed vs. unprocessed). Pay attention to how different carbohydrates affect your body, choose whole carbohydrate foods with fiber, and eat what your body needs for optimal health.

CHAPTER 15

FATS

Do you remember learning about the human cell in biology class? There was an outer layer that allowed certain things in and out of the cell, and then there were a bunch of cell "organs" (like the mitochondria) inside the cell that did all kinds of crazy things to keep us alive, moving, breathing, and thinking. Well, fat is a main component of that cell layer. It (along with its protein, vitamin, and mineral sidekicks) acts like a bouncer at a club that determines what goes in and outside the cell. It's important because if the wrong thing gets in or the right thing is not allowed in, it could mean problems for us.

Fat is also important for absorbing the fat-soluble vitamins A, E, D, and K. A little olive oil on a salad with green leafy vegetables, carrots, and sweet potatoes will help us absorb the vitamins K, E, and A in those foods. Fish, like salmon, have natural vitamin D and natural healthy fats. The combination is a match made in heaven.

Fat, like carbohydrates, is also a source of energy. While carbohydrates break down into sugar (glucose), fats break down into fatty acids in the body. Sugar and fatty acids go through a series of reactions to create energy (called ATP) that eventually drives every reaction in the body.

If Fats Are So Important, Why All of the Bad News About It?

- ☑ First, we isolated natural fats and added them in large quantities to foods that normally don't have a lot of fat. We then cooked the fats in a way that creates cancer-causing agents and is linked to heart disease (e.g., French fries).
- ☑ Second, we created "franken" fats like trans fats (more on trans fats later) that cause harm to the body. Then we stuck them in ultra-processed, addictive foods that we eat in large quantities beyond what our bodies were made to handle.
- ☑ Third, we marketed foods made with isolated and "franken" fats and made them easily accessible. Eating these foods in large quantities increases our risk for certain diseases and gives us more calories/energy than we need, thereby stressing our bodies to the point of burnout.

Storing fat is necessary for protecting the body from cold weather and falls and for those times when we can't access food over a longer stretch of time. Too much storage, though, means *excess* weight gain. Please note that weight gain is not a bad thing; it is the excess that can cause problems. There is a number that gives us a sense of whether we *may* have too much or even too little weight. It's called the body mass index.

Body Mass Index (BMI)

BMI is our weight divided by our height squared (Weight/Height^2), and it is a way to categorize specific weight and height ranges by their increased risk for disease.

— TABLE 15.1 —
BMI RATIO RANGES AND CATEGORIES

BMI RATIO (WEIGHT/HEIGHT2)	CATEGORY
<18.4	Underweight
18.5–24.9	Normal
25.0–39.9	Overweight
<40	Obese

*Underweight, overweight, and obese indicate an increased risk for disease.

BMI has received its just share of critique. Some, however, say it's a useless number. That is an unwarranted critique. The health risk associated with individuals who are categorized as underweight, overweight, or obese is just that, an increased risk. It doesn't mean that you are certain to get a disease. A fit person with a significant amount of muscle mass and a healthy diet, for example, may fall into the overweight category but may have a decreased risk for disease. At the same time, a lot of muscle does not mean an individual doesn't have an increased risk of disease. Building muscle does not make up for a poor diet.

Likewise, others may fall into the normal category but have little muscle mass and a poor diet. They may be at more risk for disease than healthy and fit individuals who fall into the overweight and obese categories. There are outlier scenarios, of course, and like the calorie recommendations and BMR (see Chapter 12), these numbers are to be used as guidance only on our way to finding what is right for our own bodies.

> **Body Mass Index (BMI)**
> BMI is a number generated by dividing weight by height squared (weight/height^2). It is used mostly to determine risk for disease. Here are the numbers.
>
> <18.4 Underweight
> 18.5–24.9 – Normal Weight
> 25.0–39.9 – Overweight
> <40–Obese
>
> To calculate your BMI, do an online search for "BMI calculator" and insert your numbers. You can also find your BMI by using Table 15.2.

Body Mass Index Table

You can calculate your own BMI, but we won't go into that here because there are convenient BMI calculators online that you can use. Search "BMI calculator" and enter your numbers. You may also use Table 15.2.

To use Table 15.2, find your height in the left-hand column labeled height. Move across to your weight (in pounds). The number at the top of the column is the BMI at that height and weight. Pounds have been rounded off.

— TABLE 15.2 —
NATIONAL INSTITUTES OF HEALTH BODY MASS INDEX TABLE[49]

BMI	19	20	21	22	23	24	25	26	27	28	29	30	31	32	33	34	35
Height (inches)							Body Weight (pounds)										
58	91	96	100	105	110	115	119	124	129	134	138	143	148	153	158	162	167
59	94	99	104	109	114	119	124	128	133	138	143	148	153	158	163	168	173
60	97	102	107	112	118	123	128	133	138	143	148	153	158	163	168	174	179
61	100	106	111	116	122	127	132	137	143	148	153	158	164	169	174	180	185
62	104	109	115	120	126	131	136	142	147	153	158	164	169	175	180	186	191
63	107	113	118	124	130	135	141	146	152	158	163	169	175	180	186	191	197
64	110	116	122	128	134	140	145	151	157	163	169	174	180	186	192	197	204
65	114	120	126	132	138	144	150	156	162	168	174	180	186	192	198	204	210
66	118	124	130	136	142	148	155	161	167	173	179	186	192	198	204	210	216
67	121	127	134	140	146	153	159	166	172	178	185	191	198	204	211	217	223
68	125	131	138	144	151	158	164	171	177	184	190	197	203	210	216	223	230
69	128	135	142	149	155	162	169	176	182	189	196	203	209	216	223	230	236
70	132	139	146	153	160	167	174	181	188	195	202	209	216	222	229	236	243
71	136	143	150	157	165	172	179	186	193	200	208	215	222	229	236	243	250
72	140	147	154	162	169	177	184	191	199	206	213	221	228	235	242	250	258
73	144	151	159	166	174	182	189	197	204	212	219	227	235	242	250	257	265
74	148	155	163	171	179	186	194	202	210	218	225	233	241	249	256	264	272
75	152	160	168	176	184	192	200	208	216	224	232	240	248	256	264	272	279
76	156	164	172	180	189	197	205	213	221	230	238	246	254	263	271	279	287

Fats had a long-time reputation for causing weight gain and causing this epidemic of obesity we are seeing around the world. More recently, carbohydrates have often been made out to be the culprit. However, neither one by themselves is to blame. It is the type and quantity that makes a difference. We reviewed healthy vs. unhealthy carbohydrates in chapter 14, now let us do the same for fats.

Are "Good" vs. "Bad" Fats a Thing?

Yes, if you define them by their health effects, like we did with carbohydrates. But again, let's just call them healthy or unhealthy.

Certain types of fat are necessary for survival and optimal health, while others allow us to survive but not necessarily thrive or achieve optimal health.

Two main groups of fat are saturated and unsaturated. Here is more information on these fats.

Saturated Fats

Saturated fats are healthy fats that are important for optimal health. They have a bad rap because we tend to consume more than our bodies need. Eating too many foods high in saturated fat can increase blood cholesterol levels (more than cholesterol itself).[50] And there is a correlation between high saturated fat consumption and increased risk of the following illnesses:
- Heart disease[51]
- Stroke[52]
- Certain cancers[53]
- Decline in brain function[54]
- Faster aging[55]

Saturated fats are found in red meats, cheese, milk (except skim), butter, many baked goods, potato chips, certain oils, and fried foods.

How Many Grams of Saturated Fats Do We Need? (Get Ready for Some More Math.)

While we need saturated fats, we don't need to eat them at all if we don't want to. Why? As long as we get our other nutrients, our bodies can make all the saturated fat they need. In fact, the RDA for saturated fat is "Not Determined."

Most of us eat saturated fats because they are hard to avoid 100%. To help us reduce our risk of heart disease associated with eating *too much* saturated fat, the American Heart Association (AHA) provides us with some guidance. They recommend that no more than 5%-6% of our calories come from saturated fat.[56] That means that the number differs for different people because we all have different caloric needs. A person with a 1,500-calorie diet will have a different recommendation from someone with a 2,500-calorie diet.

If you did your "homework" from chapter 12, you now know your BMR. Use that number to calculate your 6%. Below is an example of how to calculate 6% of calories from saturated fat for someone whose BMR is 2,000 calories a day.

1. To calculate 6% of 2,000:
    a. Multiply 6% by 2,000 = 12,000
    b. Divide 12,000 by 100 = 120 calories per day
2. To convert 120 calories to grams of fat:
    a. Recall that 1 gram of fat has 9 calories. Therefore,
    b. Divide 120 calories by 9 = 13 grams a day

> After looking up what 13 grams of saturated fat looks like, you might be shocked. Don't be discouraged though, make small changes that make a big difference. For example, you can start with something like eating a bean burrito instead of a beef burrito for lunch once a week. Or you can order the burger with a small fry instead of a large fry. It all counts!

Grams of fat is the number you will find on the nutrition facts label. See Table 15.3 to determine what 13 grams of saturated fat looks like.

Saturated Fat %DV

The USDA uses 20 grams of saturated fat daily to determine the %DV on the nutrition facts label. However, 20 grams is a little higher than the AHA recommendation of 13 grams for a person on a 2,000-calorie diet. Table 15.3 compares the %DV between these two numbers.

— TABLE 15.3 —
GRAMS OF SATURATED FAT PER SERVING FOR SEVERAL FOODS AND THEIR %DV

FOOD	SERVING SIZE	GRAMS OF SATURATED FAT	%DV PER THE NUTRITION FACTS LABEL (20 GRAMS/DAY TOTAL)	%DV PER THE AHA RECOMMENDATION (13 GRAMS/DAY TOTAL)
Beef/steak	4 ounces	9	45%	69%
Pork	4 ounces	6	30%	46%
Chicken w/ skin	4 ounces	5	25%	38%
Chicken (skinless)	4 ounces	3	15%	23%
Turkey	4 ounces	3	15%	23%
Fish	4 ounces	1	5%	8%
Eggs	1 large	2	10%	15%
Cheese	1 ounce	6	30%	46%
Milk (whole)	1 cup	5	25%	38%
Butter	1 tablespoon	7	35%	53%
Vegetable oils	1 tablespoon	2	10%	15%
Coconut oil	1 tablespoon	12	60%	92%
Potato Chips	13 chips	2	10%	15%
Ice Cream	½ Cup	6	30%	46%

*Please note that these are estimations based on multiple products. Your specific item may have more or less grams of saturated fat.

A Few Things to Note About Saturated Fats in Foods

☑ Remember to read labels and pay attention to serving sizes. The numbers above are rough estimates. You might find a brand of vanilla ice cream, for example, with 10 grams of saturated fat per ½ cup instead of the 6 grams listed in the table. And don't get me started on the caramel, chocolate, marshmallow with cookie dough type flavors!

☑ Note that chicken/turkey has less saturated fat than beef, and skinless has even less. It does

> The American Heart Association recommends no more than 13 grams of saturated fat per day for someone who eats 2,000 calories a day. Less for individuals eating less.

make a difference when you order the chicken/turkey versions of sausages, burgers, etc.
- ☑ Remember that several animal flesh products will have oils added when they are cooked, adding more saturated fat. Be aware.
- ☑ Choose canned meats that are canned with water instead of oil (the oil adds saturated fat).

How Much Is a Serving?

Per Table 15.3, if we eat four ounces of beef with one ounce of cheese, we will be at the recommended limit for the day. You will save a gram or two by purchasing leaner beef, but it's still a hefty chunk of our saturated fat %DV. But these numbers don't mean much if we don't know what a serving looks like. Table 15.4 provides this information.

— TABLE 15.4 —
WHAT A SERVING LOOKS LIKE

FOOD ITEM	SERVING SIZE	WHAT THAT LOOKS LIKE
Beef, chicken, turkey, fish/other meat	4 ounces	A little larger than the size of a deck of cards, the palm of an adult-sized hand, or the size of a *small* (not large) burger patty.
Cheese	1 ounce	4 dice put together, or one full slice used for burgers.
Butter	1 tablespoon	Use the tablespoon guide on the butter wrapping.

*Use a measuring spoon for the butter as an alternative.

Exercise: How Many Saturated Fats?

1. Using Table 15.3, take a moment to calculate how many grams of saturated fat you eat in a day below or on a separate sheet of paper. Remember to adjust based on actual serving sizes. And if you ate something like lasagna, estimate the amount of meat and cheese in each serving.

Food Item _____, grams of Saturated Fat _____

Food Item _____, grams of Saturated Fat _____

Food Item _____, grams of Saturated Fat _____

Food Item _____, grams of Saturated Fat _____

Food Item _____, grams of Saturated Fat _____

Food Item _____, grams of Saturated Fat _____

Food Item _____, grams of Saturated Fat _____

Food Item _____, grams of Saturated Fat _____

Food Item _____, grams of Saturated Fat _____

Food Item _____, grams of Saturated Fat _____

Food Item _____, grams of Saturated Fat _____

Food Item _____, grams of Saturated Fat _____

Food Item _____, grams of Saturated Fat _____

Food Item _____, grams of Saturated Fat _____

Food Item _____, grams of Saturated Fat _____

Food Item _____, grams of Saturated Fat _____

Food Item _____, grams of Saturated Fat _____

TOTAL _____

2. Compare your total to the 13 grams per day (or whatever number is recommended for your BMR).
3. If your number is less than 20 grams, you are doing well!
4. If your number is greater than 20 grams, consider replacing some higher saturated fat options with lower or no saturated fat options like lentils, beans, falafel, and tofu.

Like the carbohydrate activity, the purpose of this activity is not to stress you out about numbers but instead to create awareness of how much saturated fat is in the foods that we eat. Just being aware is enough to make healthy changes.

There is no harm in using 13 grams per day as a goal or setting your own goal, whether it's 20 grams a day or 5 grams a day. Many find success in that, and others have to work their way down slowly.

If you are starting at 50 grams a day, for example, set a goal of 40-45 grams a day and accomplish that goal just by making swaps like:

- A hamburger instead of a cheeseburger
- Chicken instead of beef
- Grilled chicken instead of fried chicken
- Beans or lentils instead of chicken

Emphasizing healthy foods and fats is another good strategy. Instead of telling yourself that you cannot have that burger and French fries, focus on telling yourself that you are going to eat the black bean burger and homemade fries that cost $2 per serving. Add some healthy fats with avocado slices for just $0.75 for half an avocado, eat some nuts for a snack, etc. More to come on healthy fats.

Is the Saturated Fat in Coconut Oil Better for You?

You may have noticed from Table 15.3 that coconut oil has more saturated fat in one tablespoon than any other item on the list. If your ear is to the ground in the health and wellness circles, you may have heard that despite its saturated fat content, coconut oil is considered much better for you than saturated fat from animal products and other plant-based oils. That's because coconut oil and coconut milk are made of medium-chain fatty acids. These are easier for the body to digest than the long-chain fatty acids found in other forms of saturated fat.

There are claims that coconut oil is good for the heart, but the evidence to support this is more anecdotal than scientific (and anecdotal evidence is important to consider). However, strong evidence suggests that coconut oil may prevent age-related neurological disorders like dementia and Alzheimer's.[57] It also has a high smoke point, which means that it doesn't burn at high temperatures and is, therefore, safer to eat when cooked. So, there are compelling reasons to choose coconut oil and coconut milk. I use coconut oil for things like baked sweet potato fries/wedges/chips and baked plantains. I also use coconut milk for cooking things like chickpea curry and rice.

If you choose to eat coconut oil, limit how much per day you eat, as it still has 130 calories per tablespoon.

Table 15.5 reviews all this information and presents some pros and cons of choosing different types of saturated fats.

— TABLE 15.5 —
THE PROS AND CONS OF EATING SATURATED FATS FROM PLANT-BASED AND ANIMAL-BASED FOODS/OILS

	SATURATED FAT FROM ANIMALS (E.G., RED MEAT, BUTTER, DAIRY, ETC.)	SATURATED FAT FROM VEGETABLE OILS (INCLUDING OILS IN FRENCH FRIES AND OTHER FRIED VEGETARIAN FOODS)	COCONUT OIL/MILK (PLANT-BASED)
PROS	✓ Fine in limited quantities	✓ Fine in limited quantities ✓ No animal cruelty ✓ Better for the planet	✓ Contain medium-chain fatty acids ✓ No animal cruelty ✓ Better for the planet ✓ Evidence suggests that it prevents neurological disorders like dementia and Alzheimer's disease
CONS	✓ Animal cruelty is a strong possibility ✓ Environmental concerns ✓ Contain long-chain fatty acids ✓ Increases cholesterol in the blood ✓ Increased consumption correlated with heart disease, and cancer ✓ Can cause excess weight gain in large quantities	✓ Contains long-chain fatty acids ✓ Increases cholesterol in the blood ✓ Increased consumption correlated with heart disease, cancer, and kidney disease ✓ Can cause excess weight gain in large quantities	✓ Can cause excess weight gain in large quantities

What About Cholesterol?

Cholesterol is an important nutrient for the body and is found only in animal products like eggs, meat, poultry, dairy, some shellfish, butter, and cheese. Without cholesterol, our cells would collapse, reactions important to the body wouldn't occur, we wouldn't be able to form vitamin D, and our brains would not function well. Remember the outer wall of the cell that fat is important for? Well, cholesterol also forms a part of that wall.

Cholesterol is not fat and does not have any calories. However, too much cholesterol does make some contributions to plaque buildup in the blood vessels, which contributes to heart disease and stroke risk.

> Eating saturated fats can increase cholesterol more than eating cholesterol itself.

No plant-based foods have cholesterol. That's right, potato chips and French fries do not have cholesterol. However, they have saturated fat (see Table 15.3), which may increase blood cholesterol levels more than cholesterol itself.

Healthy (HDL) vs. Unhealthy (LDL) Cholesterol

Two types of cholesterol in our bodies are high-density lipoproteins (HDL) and low-density lipoproteins (LDL). When we get our blood work done at the doctor's office, we want to see a high HDL cholesterol (above 60) and a low LDL cholesterol (under 100). Here is why:

- ☑ **LDL cholesterol** goes through the body, making a mess of things. It makes cholesterol deposits in the blood vessels and clog things up, making it hard for blood to pass through. This can lead to a heart attack and/or stroke. See Table 15.6 for foods that increase LDL cholesterol.
- ☑ **HDL cholesterol** goes through the body, cleaning things up. See Table 15.6 for foods that increase HDL cholesterol.

— TABLE 15.6 —
FOODS THAT INCREASE HDL AND LDL CHOLESTEROL

FOODS THAT INCREASE "HEALTHY" CHOLESTEROL (HDL)	FOODS THAT INCREASE "UNHEALTHY" CHOLESTEROL (LDL)
• Oatmeal • Fatty fish, like salmon and tuna • Almonds and other nuts • Avocado • Olive oil • Fruits (esp. apples and pears) • Vegetables • Beans • Lentils	• Foods high in saturated fat (see Table 15.3) • Red meat • Pork • Processed meats like sausage, bacon, hot dogs and salami • Butter and cheese • Fried foods • Potato chips • Cookies and cakes

What About the Cholesterol in Shrimp?

Shrimp has cholesterol, and evidence suggests that the cholesterol in shrimp may increase LDL cholesterol in our blood. It also suggests that it increases HDL cholesterol.[58] It is a low-calorie, high-quality protein source with healthy omega-3 fats and virtually no saturated fat. Despite these benefits, shrimp does elevate LDL cholesterol and should be eaten in moderation.

What About the Cholesterol in Eggs?

Are you confused as to whether you should eat eggs? You are not alone. Eggs are arguably the most controversial of all the whole foods. There are some very compelling reasons to eat eggs. And there are some compelling reasons not to eat eggs, especially if you have heart disease or are at risk for stroke.

Table 15.7 provides some pros and cons for you to decide for yourself if eggs are right for you, but my recommendation is:

☑ Limit eggs to two a day if you aren't eating several other sources of saturated fat and cholesterol.

☑ If you are eating several other sources of saturated fat/cholesterol, have heart disease, or have an increased risk for stroke, no more than one egg a day.

☑ The healthiest way to eat eggs is to eat them hard-boiled or baked to avoid adding saturated fat.

— TABLE 15.7 —
THE PROS AND CONS OF EATING EGGS

PROS	✓ Contains choline which is important for brain function and is hard to find in other food sources ✓ Contains vitamins D and A, which are also very important and hard to find in other food sources ✓ They are a very low-calorie source of protein and may aid in weight and blood sugar management
CONS	✓ High in cholesterol ✓ Increased consumption is associated with an increased risk of cardiovascular disease in individuals with other health conditions[59]

Trans Fats

Trans fats (also known as partially hydrogenated oils) are fats created in a lab. Remember when advertisers told us to eat margarine instead of butter because it was better for the heart back in the day? That margarine was made with trans fats. It turned out that trans fats are worse for our heart health than the saturated fats they were supposed to replace as a healthier alternative.

In fact, trans fats made in factories are so bad that they have been banned in the United States. That is quite the feat, given all the chemicals and junk that the government allows companies to put in our food. A few foods naturally have trans fats in very small quantities, but for the most part, you don't have to worry about trans fats being added to foods.

I mention trans fats because they offer an example of what happens often in the food industry. That is:

1. Food manufacturers create an alternative to a food item that is harmful when eaten in large quantities.
2. They tell us the new ingredient is healthy.
3. We trust them and eat the food in large quantities.
4. Years later, we find out that the "healthier alternative" is worse than the original.

I don't blame us for believing them. We trust that our fellow human beings will have our best interests at heart. Unfortunately, we have to put that trust on hold when it comes to new foods on the market. Oftentimes, the almighty dollar wins over concerns about our health when it comes to our food system. Even the most well-intentioned food creators find it hard to create products that are healthy per our definition of healthy, which is to cause no harm. That is because to be as profitable as possible on the supermarket shelves, food requires a lot of processing and preservatives.

> New food concoctions (e.g., meat substitutes, artificial sweeteners, GMOs, etc.) are placed on the market and often promoted as healthy alternatives or at the very least, safe to eat. These claims are made even though the new product typically is not tested for long-term health effects. These food companies basically test on anyone willing to believe their claim and eat their products.

Food companies make a whole lot of money during what I call their guinea pig phase. When we find out their products are not good for us, they may take them off the market… or not, depending on if the government deems them dangerous *enough*. And we know that if the government yanks something off the market, it is probably as bad as it can get.

The fact that they took trans fats off of the market speaks a lot as to how dangerous they were to our health. Yet, for a long time, we ate them as if they were better for us. Imagine that a substance is literally killing us, and we are convinced that we are helping ourselves. It is THE story of our food system.

When you read the ingredients lists, you might see something called hydrogenated oils. This is often found in peanut butter. These are different from *partially* hydrogenated oils (or trans fats) because they are "fully" hydrogenated. They are considered to be safer than partially hydrogenated oils, so the government allows food manufacturers to use them. However, as I mentioned before, just because the government allows them, that does not mean that they are safe. Avoid hydrogenated oils if you can.

Unsaturated Fats: "The Good Fats"

Let's talk about the fats that are often referred to as the "good" fats or unsaturated fats. There are 2 main types of unsaturated fats:
1. Monounsaturated
2. Polyunsaturated

Monounsaturated Fats: Omega-9's "The Really Good Fats"

Research suggests that monounsaturated fats play an important anti-inflammatory role and a role in preventing cancer.[60] Our bodies can make monounsaturated fats, however, they are important for us to incorporate into our diets to help us maximize their health benefits. A useful technique for incorporating these into our diet is to consider making some swaps. See Table 15.8 for some delicious and easy swaps.

— TABLE 15.8 —
MONOUNSATURATED FAT FOR SATURATED FAT SWAPS

INSTEAD OF (SATURATED FAT)...	TRY (MONOUNSATURATED FAT)...
Cheese or meat on your salad	Nuts or avocados
Cheese on your burger	Avocado slices
Ham, bologna, or salami sandwich	Peanut (or almond) butter sandwich
Potato chips	Sunflower or pumpkin seeds
Ranch dressing	Olive oil, vinegar, and honey mixture
Vegetable oil	Avocado oil (It's more expensive but can be a gift that you request. It is also important to use in limited quantities for health and savings purposes)

A Few Foods with Monounsaturated Fats

- Almonds
- Avocadoes

- Avocado oil (for cooking)
- Peanuts
- Peanut or almond butter
- Pecans
- Pumpkin seeds
- Sesame seeds
- Uncooked olive oil

There is no specific recommendation for monounsaturated fats. However, one to two swaps from Table 15.8 can play a role in improving our health.

Polyunsaturated Fats: Omega-3's "The Other Really Good Fats"

Unlike monounsaturated fats, we cannot make omega-3 fats ourselves. This means that we must get them in our diet.

They are largely found in fish and several plant-based foods like olives, avocados, and nuts. This means that we get an omega-9 and omega-3 bundle. Research suggests that omega-3 consumption improves heart, eye, and brain health and helps prevent cancer.[61] There is also evidence that they reduce inflammation and arthritis pain.[62]

Omega-3 Fat Recommendation

Omega-3 fats are not included on the nutrition facts label, but because they are essential, there is a daily recommendation. That recommendation is 1.6 grams per day for males 9-70 years of age and 1.1 per day for females who are not pregnant or lactating between 9-70 years of age.[63]

Again, this number is not the be-all and end-all, but it provides us with a reference point to work from. See Table 15.9 for foods with omega-3s and quantities to ensure you are getting your omega-3s in!

— TABLE 15.9 —
SOURCES OF OMEGA-3 FATS AND THEIR %DV

FOOD	SERVING SIZE	GRAMS OF OMEGA-3 FAT	%DV PER THE NUTRITION FACTS LABEL (NOT PROVIDED)	%DV PER THE ADEQUATE INTAKE RECOMMENDATION (1.6 GRAMS/DAY TOTAL)
Salmon	4 ounces	2.5	–	156%
Chia Seeds	1 tablespoon	2.5	–	156%
Walnuts	1 ounce	2.5	–	156%
Flaxseed (ground)	1 tablespoon	1.8	–	113%
Sardines	4 ounces	1.7	–	106%
Soybeans	½ cup	0.8	–	50%
Kidney Beans	½ cup	0.5	–	31%
Avocado	1 whole	0.2	–	12%
Brussels Sprouts (cooked)	1 cup	0.1	–	6%

*Most fish types, beans, nuts, and seeds have omega-3s. The ones mentioned in this table have the highest amounts. Also note that some foods are fortified with omega 3's.

One serving of fish (wild-caught responsibly is best if you have it in your budget) is an easy way to incorporate the omega-3s we need into our food routines. If you don't like fish, are conscious of the environment/animal treatment, or don't want to spend half your paycheck on wild-caught versions, plant-based versions of omega-3s are great.

Most plant-based foods with omega-3s contain the ALA form of omega-3s. Some of that ALA is converted to EPA and DHA (the omega-3s found in fish and seaweed). All three forms of omega-3s offer important health benefits. If you are vegetarian, eating vegetables, beans, nuts, and seeds regularly is sufficient to ensure you are getting your recommended amount for the day.

Chia seeds and flaxseeds are especially easy ways to incorporate omega-3s into our diets. Flaxseeds can be added to soups, sauces, oatmeal, and other hot cereals. Chia and flaxseeds also have fiber, so they pack a powerful punch for health. They both go for about $5.00-$10.00 for about 15-25 servings or about $0.35 per serving, depending on the brand. I always recommend organic if you can get it.

A Note About Flaxseeds

Flaxseeds must be ground with a grinder to access their omega-3 fats. Purchase the whole flaxseed and grind them yourself only when ready to eat them. This is important because the fats go bad faster once you grind them. You can use a coffee or spice grinder to grind your flaxseeds, and you can find grinders starting at $10.00. This is another nice gift to ask for; a bag of organic flaxseeds with a grinder is the perfect gift.

What About Omega-3 Supplements?

If you are eating vegetables, beans, nuts, seeds, and other foods regularly, you will get the omega-3s that you need and the health benefits that come with them. Omega-3 supplements are not necessary for optimal health. However, if you are suffering from arthritis pain or some other inflammatory conditions, they can help alleviate symptoms.

Polyunsaturated Fats: Omega-6s, the "Good Fats"

These are often referred to as "good fats." The problem is that they are often found in foods high in saturated fat and sugar (like baked goods, potato chips, and fried foods). Therefore, we eat much more than we need, which, as you know, puts stress on the body. In this case, evidence suggests that the large influx of omega-6s can cause inflammation and heart disease.[64]

Table 15.10 summarizes the fats we have discussed so far, and Table 15.11 lists the sources of these fats.

— TABLE 15.10 —
FATS THAT WE GET TOO MANY OF AND FATS THAT WE DON'T GET ENOUGH OF

	MONO-UNSATURATED FATS (OMEGA-9S)	POLY-UNSATURATED FATS (OMEGA-3S)	POLY-UNSATURATED FATS (OMEGA-6S)	SATURATED FATS (LONG-CHAIN)	SATURATED FATS (MEDIUM-CHAIN)
Most don't get enough	X	X			
Most get too many			X	X	X

— TABLE 15.11 —
COMMON SOURCES OF FATS WITH THEIR MOST PREVALENT FAT CONTENT

FOOD ITEM	MONO-UNSATURATED FATS (OMEGA-9S)	POLY-UNSATURATED FATS (OMEGA-3S)	POLY-UNSATURATED FATS (OMEGA 6S)	SATURATED FATS (LONG-CHAIN)	SATURATED FATS (MEDIUM-CHAIN)
Avocado	X	X			
Salmon		X			
Nuts (esp. walnuts)	X	X	X		
Flax Seeds		X			
Chia seeds		X			
Olive oil		X			
Spinach		X			
Kale		X			
Brussels Sprouts		X			
Beans (esp. Kidney)		X			
Coconut oil					X
Beef/steak			X	X	
Pork			X	X	
Chicken			X	X	
Turkey				X	
Cheese				X	
Butter				X	
Eggs		X	X	X	
Potato chips			X	X	
Milk (Whole, 2%, 1%)				X	
Baked goods			X	X	

*Choose foods that contain the first two columns.

Is Fish Good for Me?

Fish has omega 3's and vitamin D and is a low-calorie source of protein. Unfortunately, pollution has taken its toll on our water friends, so along with the wonderful health benefits of fish, you also will get some of those pollutants. That is why a common recommendation is no more than one to two servings (four ounces per serving) a week. Recall that four ounces is a little bigger than the size of a deck of cards.

Some fish are raised on fish farms, and others are caught in the wild. Table 15.12 lists the pros and cons of each so you can decide which is right for you. If you read the pros and cons of each and find that it's not worth it, it is ok not to eat fish as the nutrients can be obtained from plant-based sources, and it is better for the planet.

— TABLE 15.12 —
THE PROS AND CONS OF FARM-RAISED AND WILD-CAUGHT FISH

	FARM-RAISED FISH	WILD-CAUGHT FISH
PROS	✓ Contains Omega-3 fats and Vitamin D ✓ Low-calorie protein source	✓ Contains Omega-3 fats and Vitamin D ✓ Low-calorie protein source
CONS	✓ Environmental concerns ✓ Animal cruelty likely ✓ More likely to have diseases ✓ May contain antibiotics to treat those diseases ✓ Contains mercury	✓ More expensive ✓ May not be sustainable depending on the fish ✓ Contains mercury

What About Oils?

There are several types of oils and cooking fats, and everybody seems to have something to say about which is best and which is the worst. That is why I will give this tip; limit the amount of oil you eat and cook with. Oils are processed foods high in calories and fat, and many of them are associated with weight gain and heart disease. The biggest problem with oils, aside from the calorie load, is that their chemical structure changes when we cook with them, making them harmful to our health. Fats like butter, lard, and tallow that come from animals should also be limited. Again, limiting how much oil/fat we use and cook with is the key.

Certain oils, like avocado oil, have a high smoke point which means they can tolerate a lot of heat without changing their structure. They are, therefore, better for cooking. Unfortunately, they can be very expensive, and they, too, are high in calories like the others (about 120 calories per tablespoon). If you cook with oils or other fats, stick with cooking methods that don't require a lot, like, sautéing, baking, roasting, and steaming (see chapter 1).

Smoke point = the temperature at which oil begins to burn.

Pure vs. Extra Virgin Olive Oil

I often get questions about the difference between pure and extra virgin oil. Table 15.13 provides information about the difference.

— TABLE 15.13 —
PROS AND CONS OF PURE AND EXTRA VIRGIN OLIVE OIL

	PURE OLIVE OIL	EXTRA-VIRGIN OLIVE OIL
PROS	✓ Better for cooking at low temperatures ✓ Less expensive	✓ Minimal processing ✓ Higher in Omega 3s ✓ Better when eaten raw (dressings and dips)
CONS	✓ More processing ✓ Less omega-3s and plant nutrients (like antioxidants and polyphenols) ✓ Should not be used for frying	✓ Not recommended for cooking ✓ Usually more expensive

Choosing a healthy oil is hard, especially if you are on a budget. No matter what you choose, though, be sure to limit how much you eat from a health and savings perspective. I have several oils in my pantry. I use avocado oil for sautéing. Pure olive oil, or avocado oil for baking/roasting. I use coconut oil for things like sweet potato fries and plantains and extra virgin olive oil for making salad dressings and dips.

They cost more than vegetable or canola oil (unless you ask for oils as gifts), but I don't use them a lot, so they last a long time. I bought a large tub of organic extra virgin coconut oil for about $20.00, and a year later, I still have it in my pantry.

Again, the best thing to do for optimal health and for the wallet is to choose cooking methods that don't require a lot of oil or fat. Baking/roasting, grilling (without the grill marks), steaming, and sautéing are all great options.

> For a heart-healthy swap, replace butter for spreading and salad dressings like ranch, which are high in saturated fat, with extra virgin olive oil.

Fats—The Takeaway

Fats are important for optimal health. Plant-based fats found in foods like nuts, seeds, beans, and vegetables are great healthy sources of fats that help with brain and heart health, weight management, aging, inflammation, and they have other health benefits.

Animal-based fats found in foods like beef, butter, tallow, and whole milk have saturated fat, which when eaten in large quantities, can cause weight gain and heart problems.

Oils are fats extracted from plants. Some oils provide more health benefits than others; however, limiting your oil intake altogether is a good idea for optimal health.

We discussed carbohydrates and fats in detail. Let's move on to proteins.

CHAPTER 16

PROTEINS

When we eat protein, it breaks down into amino acids. These amino acids then get to building all of the things we need to stay alive. If you have hair, nails, muscle, bones, blood, hormones, enzymes, and even cells, then you have eaten protein. Because proteins (amino acids) make up the infrastructure of our bodies, they are known as the body's building blocks.

Complete vs. Incomplete Proteins.

Nine amino acids are considered essential. That means we can't produce them ourselves, so we must get them from our food.

Non-essential amino acids are amino acids we can make ourselves, so we don't have to get them through food. Table 16.1 lists the nonessential and essential amino acids.

— TABLE 16.1 —
LIST OF NON-ESSENTIAL AND ESSENTIAL AMINO ACIDS

NON-ESSENTIAL AMINO ACIDS	ESSENTIAL AMINO ACIDS
Alanine	Histidine
Arginine	Isoleucine
Asparagine	Leucine
Aspartic Acid	Lysine

NON-ESSENTIAL AMINO ACIDS	ESSENTIAL AMINO ACIDS
Cysteine	Methionine
Glutamic acid	Phenylalanine
Glutamine	Threonine
Glycine	Tryptophan
Proline	Valine
Serine	
Tyrosine	

Complete Proteins
Foods that contain all nine essential amino acids.

Incomplete Proteins
Foods that do not contain all nine essential amino acids.

Complete proteins are foods that have all nine essential amino acids. Incomplete proteins do not contain all nine essential amino acids. This does not mean that complete proteins are healthier for you. In fact, incomplete proteins have more fiber, vitamins, minerals, and antioxidants than most complete proteins (see Table 16.2).

Where Can You Find Complete Proteins?

— TABLE 16.2 —
LIST OF COMPLETE AND INCOMPLETE PROTEINS

COMPLETE PROTEINS	INCOMPLETE PROTEINS
Fish	Vegetables
Poultry	Fruit
Meat	Beans
Fish	Lentils
Seafood	Nuts
Egg	Seeds
All dairy products	Whole grains (rice, wheat and oats)
Quinoa	

*Note that quinoa is one of the only plant-based complete proteins.

Most plant-based foods are incomplete proteins. For example, rice does not contain lysine, but beans do. Beans do not have enough methionine, but rice does, so beans and rice are the perfect food pairing.

Vegans and vegetarians do not need to stress about incomplete proteins as long as they eat various plant-based foods. There are some things to be aware of if vegetarianism or veganism is your preference—incomplete proteins aren't one of them.

How Much Protein Do You Need?

Not as much as you might think. The RDA for protein for healthy people between the ages of 19 and 70 who are not pregnant or lactating is 46 grams per day for females and 56 grams per day for males.

This recommendation varies widely per individual, but most people (especially carnivores) eat more protein than they need, especially if they do not exercise much. Another recommendation specific to body weight can get us closer to our specific needs.

* * *

Protein Recommendation Specific to Body Weight=
0.36 grams of protein per pound per day

* * *

This number is for someone who does not get much exercise or has no other medical conditions that change protein requirements. Yes, there's more math here, and whenever math is involved, you know I will provide examples, so here it is.

* * *

Examples Using RDA Specific to Body Weight (i.e., 0.36 grams/day)
1. How many grams of protein are recommended for a 150-pound person with no medical conditions and does minimal exercise?

Answer:
Multiply 150 pounds times 0.36, and you get 54 grams of protein daily.

150 pounds * 0.36 grams = 54 grams per day

2. Now calculate how many grams of protein are recommended for your weight if you have low physical activity levels.

Answer:
Your Weight Here: _____ pounds

Multiply your weight by (0.36) grams

= _____ **grams per day is your protein requirement.**

* * *

How to Determine if You Are Including This Amount of Protein in Your Diet?

- ☑ Use Table 16.3 to calculate approximately how many grams of protein you eat daily. The table provides grams *per serving* for commonly eaten foods.
- ☑ The nutrition facts label does not have a percent daily value (%DV) for protein, but that's ok; it has grams of protein per serving, and that's all you need.
- ☑ Beware of the health halo effect. The health halo effect is when a particular food is perceived as healthy for one reason or another, even if it may not be. For example, when many of us see the word "protein" on a package, we tend to think

> Just because a food product has the word "protein" on the package, that does not mean that it is good for you.

it is healthy. Don't believe the hype. Trust your ability to read the nutrition fact label and ingredients list from Chapter 13.

— TABLE 16.3 —
GRAMS OF PROTEIN AND %DV PER SERVING FOR SEVERAL FOODS

FOOD	SERVING SIZE	GRAMS OF PROTEIN	%DV PER THE NUTRITION FACTS LABEL (NOT PROVIDED)	%DV PER THE RDA RECOMMENDATION (56 GRAMS/DAY TOTAL)
Chicken, Turkey, Fish, Beef/steak, or Pork	4-ounces	24 grams	–	42%
Greek Yogurt	¾ cup	16 grams	–	28%
Cottage Cheese	½ cup	12 grams	–	21%
Lentils	½ cup cooked	9 grams	–	16%
Tofu	3 ounces	9 grams	–	16%
Yogurt (non-Greek)	¾ cup	8 grams	–	14%
Beans	½ cup cooked	8 grams	–	14%
Quinoa	1 cup cooked	8 grams	–	14%
Eggs	1 large	6 grams	–	10%
Nuts	¼ cup	6 grams	–	10%
Oatmeal	1 cup cooked	5 grams	–	9%
Green peas	½ cup cooked	4 grams	–	7%
Brown rice	½ cup cooked	3 grams	–	5%
Raw kale	1 cup raw	2 grams	–	4%

*Please note that these are estimations based on multiple products. Your specific food item may have more or less grams of protein per serving.

Eating more protein than we need can cause a problem if:
- ☑ We eat significantly more than is necessary. Over time, too much protein can overwork the kidneys and cause kidney disease.
- ☑ The protein comes from foods that are also high in saturated fat, like beef, cheese, sausages, bacon, and fried meats.
- ☑ The proteins come from processed foods, like protein bars with chemicals, sugar, and/or artificial sweeteners.

Is It Better to Get Protein from Animal Products?

Plant-based *whole foods* will always be the best (and most affordable) way to get most nutrients, including protein. It may seem like it's easier to get protein from animal products from Table 16.3, but there are several downsides to eating meat that you won't have to worry about when you eat plants (see Chapter 15). That is, of course, unless unhealthy things are done to them.

Some animal products, like Greek yogurt, cottage cheese, and eggs, are a great way to get protein because they are lean and nutrient-packed. If they are organic and local, even better.

For most of us, the following items are enough to get all the protein we need in a day:

- ☑ 1 cup of oatmeal with ¼ cup of nuts
- ☑ 1 cup of lentils with ½ cup of rice
- ☑ 1 cup of quinoa with 1 cup of Brussels sprouts and 3 ounces of tofu.
- ☑ For B12 (which almost exclusively comes from animal products), you can add a serving of cottage cheese or Greek yogurt.

What About Protein Powders?

I like to call myself a protein purest because I recommend getting proteins from food only, not powders and supplements if you can. Here's why:

- ☑ Most people don't need protein powders (even those who exercise) because most of us already get more than enough in our diets. If you are doing intense exercise, you will need to add more protein to your diet, but it doesn't need to be in the form of powders.
- ☑ Like we found out with sugar, we just don't know how isolating a nutrient and eating it in large quantities will impact our health over the long term.

- ☑ When you isolate a nutrient, it doesn't synergize with the other nutrients in the food. You, therefore, miss out on the health benefits of those other nutrients.
- ☑ Several protein powders contain added sweeteners, thickeners, artificial flavors, and other chemicals.
- ☑ The FDA does not regulate them, so the claims made about the contents may not be true.
- ☑ They are very expensive and useless for most people.

Which Protein Powder Should I Choose?

If you have a medical condition or other condition where you must use protein powder, use the following criteria:

- ☑ It should only have one ingredient that you recognize (no more than three ingredients, and you should recognize all of them).
- ☑ Avoid added sweeteners, flavors, thickeners, and other chemicals.
- ☑ Find a company that you trust.

What About Protein Bars?

Most protein bars are expensive and are not worth the price because they are often as bad as or worse than candy bars when it comes to nutrition. This is an item I recommend avoiding. Or, if you do eat them, use your knowledge of the nutrition facts label and ingredients list to make a healthier choice.

There are some bars out there that are not necessarily promoted as protein bars that are great healthy snacks. The ones with dates and nuts as the main ingredients, for example, are fantastic and delicious. Larabar is one of my favorite brands to eat, and I recommend it if it is in your budget. They cost less than $8.00 for a box of 6 (or about $1.30 per bar) or less than $2.00 for an individual bar.

The Most Affordable and Healthiest Proteins

It just so happens that the most affordable proteins are the most nutrient-packed. Table 16.5 provides a list of the many proteins that are readily available at an affordable cost.

— TABLE 16.5 —
THE MOST AFFORDABLE AND HEALTHIEST PROTEINS

FOOD	SERVING SIZE	COST PER FAMILY OF 4	COST PER SERVING
Lentils	½ cup cooked	$2.00	$0.50
Beans	½ cup cooked	$2.00	$0.50
Chickpeas	½ cup cooked	$2.00	$0.50
Split peas and green peas	½ cup cooked	$2.00	$0.50
Quinoa	½ cup cooked	$3.00	$0.75
Eggs	1 large	$4.00	$0.35
Nuts	¼ cup	$4.00	$1.00
Kale	1 cup raw	$2.00	$0.50
Greek yogurt	6 ounces	$5.00	$1.25
Cottage cheese	½ cup	$1.50	$1.50
Fish	3-ounces	$6.00	$1.50
Chicken or turkey	3-ounces	$8.00	$2.00

Protein—The Takeaway

You are more than likely getting enough protein in your diet to meet your daily protein needs. Protein from plant-based whole foods are preferable sources of protein because they contain fiber and other nutrients that promote optimal health.

CHAPTER 17

VITAMINS, MINERALS AND PHYTONUTRIENTS

Vitamins, minerals, and phytonutrients are micronutrients and they are harder to see with the naked eye, but that does not make them any less important than the macronutrients that we can see easily (i.e., carbohydrates, fats, and proteins). In fact, we cannot harvest energy from carbohydrates, fats, and proteins without vitamins, minerals, and phytochemicals. This is why if we are missing any, we can become ill. Likewise, if we get all the nutrients we need, we experience tremendous health benefits. They are like invisible superheroes protecting us from hurt, harm, and danger.

Phytonutrients

You know that vitamins and minerals are a big deal, so allow me first to shine some light onto their lesser-known counterparts, phytonutrients. Phytonutrients are a generic term for a host of plant nutrients. They include antioxidants. You might be familiar with some of the names of certain phytonutrients/antioxidants in Table 17.1. The phytonutrients listed in Table 17.1 are the tip of the iceberg. Several other known (and unknown) phytonutrients war on our behalf once they enter our bodies.

> Phytonutrients are powerhouse, disease-fighting nutrients that are found in plant-based whole foods.

— TABLE 17.1 —
PHYTONUTRIENT SOURCES AND HEALTH BENEFITS

PHYTONUTRIENT	SOURCES	HEALTH BENEFITS
Flavonoids[65]	✓ Leafy vegetables, blackberries, cherries, apples, grapefruit, oranges, limes, cocoa, dark chocolate, green tea, parsley and other fruits and veggies	✓ Cancer prevention ✓ Heart disease prevention ✓ Anti-inflammatory ✓ Anti-viral ✓ Anti-allergic
Carotenoids (e.g., beta-carotene, lycopene, and lutein)[66]	✓ Apricots, bell peppers, broccoli, cantaloupe, carrots, guava, grapefruit, leafy greens, mangos, pumpkin, sweet potatoes, watermelon, winter squash and most green and orange fruits and veggies	✓ Eye health (yes, it is true, carrots are good for the eyes) ✓ Skin protection ✓ Cancer prevention ✓ Heart disease prevention
Catechins[67]	✓ Green tea, apples, cacao, grapes, and berries.	✓ Cancer prevention ✓ Heart disease prevention ✓ Neurodegenerative disease like Alzheimer's disease prevention ✓ Anti-obesity activity

These phytonutrients are to vitamins and minerals what Robin is to Batman. One might even argue that they are Batmen themselves, just Batmen who do different things. Either way, they need each other to ensure we are healthy and safe. The best way to get them working optimally together is through food (and drinks like green tea). Supplements are helpful if one has a nutrient deficiency or specific symptoms (e.g., curcumin supplements may help with arthritic pain). However, they are not as good at alleviating symptoms and preventing disease as an unprocessed plant-based, healthy diet and exercise.

> Vitamins and minerals work with phytonutrients in food to protect us from pollutants, stress and other harms that come and threaten our health. You will not find that type of teamwork in supplements.

Passing on fruits, vegetables, and other whole plant-based food is like having superheroes hanging around to protect us and us saying to the superheroes, "I'm good; I think I will go with the criminal." Let's start choosing the superheroes.

Micronutrients on The Nutrition Facts Label

Five micronutrients are on the nutrition facts label: potassium, vitamin D, calcium, iron, and sodium. Sodium is one micronutrient that we tend to consume too much of (see Chapter 18). Most of us don't get enough of the other four micronutrients listed. In fact, that is why they were chosen to be represented there. This chapter will highlight these and several other micronutrients and how we can ensure we get all our superhero powers through food.

Vitamin D

If you asked me which vitamin is most important for our diets, I would say all of them. But if I had to choose one to emphasize, it would be vitamin D, hands down. Not because its role is more important than the others but because it can be difficult to incorporate into our diets, and countless diseases are associated with low vitamin D levels. Diseases like cancer, cardiovascular disease, multiple sclerosis, schizophrenia, and depression are all linked to vitamin D deficiency.[68]

There are some foods that have Vitamin D but an important way to get vitamin D is through sun exposure. A student asked me, "How does the sun put vitamin D into our bodies?" Which I thought was a brilliant question. The sun does not "put" vitamin D in the body. Instead, the UV rays from the sun convert inactive vitamin D molecules into active vitamin D molecules that then go to work. And where do inactive vitamin D molecules come from? Recall from Chapter 15 that cholesterol is the base molecule necessary to form vitamin D. In other words, if there is no cholesterol, there is no vitamin D. It all works together.

Recommended Amount of Vitamin D

The RDA for Vitamin D is 15 micrograms (mcg) per day. Table 17.2 provides a few affordable ways to meet this requirement. Also, to find out if a packaged food has vitamin D, we can look at the nutrition facts label for the %DV (see Figure 6). Here is another opportunity for you to apply the information you have about the %DV.

Vitamin D 2mcg	10%
Calcium 260mg	20%
Iron 6mg	35%
Potassium 240mg	6%

- The % Daily Value (DV) tells you how much a nutrient in a serving of food contributes to a daily diet. 2,000 calories a day is used for general nutrition advice.

Figure 6. Nutrition Facts Label %DV example

— TABLE 17.2 —
AFFORDABLE SOURCES OF VITAMIN D AND THEIR PERCENT DAILY VALUE (%DV)

VITAMIN D SOURCE	VITAMIN D PERCENT DAILY VALUE (% DV) PER SERVING
Canned Salmon	25% per 3 ounces
Plant-based milk	20-30% per cup (depending on type–read labels)
Tuna fish	10% per 3 ounces
Milk	15% per cup
Fortified orange juice	10% per cup
Eggs	6%-30% per egg (depending on type – read the labels)
15–20 minutes of sun without cloud cover or sunscreen	A few times a week can generate almost all of the vitamin D we need.[69]

Vitamin D Supplements

I don't recommend supplements often, but because vitamin D is more difficult to find in our food, I recommend a supplement for those more susceptible to vitamin deficiency, including:

- ☑ The elderly
- ☑ People who have problems absorbing fat

- ☑ Those who live in colder climates or have difficulties getting sun
- ☑ Those with low vitamin D levels per their lab work from the doctor

If you have any medical conditions, speak with your doctor first before taking any supplements.

A Note on Multivitamins

Research suggests that there is no harm in taking multivitamins. Research also suggests, however, that it does not do much good either unless you have a specific nutrient deficiency or need. Some people take supplements to make sure that their vitamin and mineral bases are covered, and that is fine. However, a good supplement by a trustworthy company can be expensive, and like protein powders, it can be a waste of money. Tables 17.3 and 17.4 provide a tastier and more affordable way to ensure you are getting your nutrients – that is, through food.

Vitamins and Minerals from Food Instead of Supplements

Eating a few items from each category in Tables 17.3 and 17.4 can help ensure you get all these nutrients and eliminate the need for supplements (unless you have a deficiency or a health condition). Eating lots of fruits and vegetables with different colors is another way to get these nutrients without having to keep tabs. Each food has multiple nutrients, so eating something like a sweet potato will provide potassium, vitamin A, certain B vitamins, and phytonutrients.

* * *

Vitamins and Minerals Activity

1. Skim through the foods listed in Tables 17.3 and 17.4.
2. Highlight the foods that you currently eat.
3. Circle the foods that you don't eat but think you might want to incorporate into your diet.
4. List the foods that you circled here or on a separate sheet of paper and try to incorporate them into your diet:

_____

_____

_____

_____

_____

_____

The charts incorporate things like pork and beef. If you choose to eat those, eat in moderation. Remember that plant-based foods are the best sources of vitamins and minerals due to their phytochemicals and mountains of evidence that they promote optimal health and are better for the planet.

— TABLE 17.3 —
VITAMIN FUNCTIONS, SOURCES, AND DAILY NEEDS (VALUE)[70]

VITAMIN	FUNCTION	SOURCES	DAILY VALUE
Biotin	• Energy storage • Protein, carbohydrate, and fat metabolism	• Avocados • Cauliflower • Eggs • Fruits (e.g., raspberries) • Liver • Pork • Salmon • Whole grains	30 mcg

VITAMIN	FUNCTION	SOURCES	DAILY VALUE
Choline	• Brain development Cell signaling • Lipid (fat) transport and metabolism • Liver function • Muscle movement Nerve function • Normal metabolism	• Beans and peas • Egg yolks • Fish (e.g., cod and salmon) • Liver (e.g., beef and chicken) • Milk • Nuts • Salmon • Soy foods • Vegetables (e.g., broccoli, cauliflower, spinach)	550 mg
Folate/Folic Acid (B9)	• Prevention of birth defects • Protein metabolism • Red blood cell formation	• Asparagus • Avocados • Beans and peas • Enriched grain products (e.g., bread, cereal, pasta, rice) • Green leafy vegetables (e.g., spinach) • Oranges and orange juice	400 mcg DFE**
Niacin (B3)	• Cholesterol production • Conversion of food into energy • Digestion • Nervous system function	• Beans • Beef • Enriched grain products (e.g., bread, cereal, pasta, rice) • Nuts • Pork • Poultry • Seafood • Whole grains	16 mg**
Pantothenic Acid (B5)	• Conversion of food into energy • Fat metabolism • Hormone production • Nervous system function • Red blood cell formation	• Avocados • Beans and peas • Broccoli • Eggs • Milk • Mushrooms • Poultry • Seafood • Sweet potatoes • Whole grains • Yogurt	5 mg
Riboflavin (B2)	• Conversion of food into energy • Growth and development • Red blood cell formation	• Eggs • Enriched grain products (e.g., bread, cereal, pasta, rice) • Meat • Milk • Mushrooms • Poultry • Seafood (e.g., oysters) • Spinach	1.3 mg

VITAMIN	FUNCTION	SOURCES	DAILY VALUE
Thiamin (B1)	• Conversion of food into energy • Nervous system function	• Beans and peas • Enriched grain products (e.g., bread, cereal, pasta, rice) • Nuts • Pork • Sunflower seeds • Whole grains	1.2 mg
Vitamin A	• Growth and development • Immune function • Red blood cell formation • Reproduction • Skin and bone formation • Vision	• Cantaloupe • Carrots • Dairy products • Eggs • Fortified cereals • Green leafy vegetables (e.g., spinach and broccoli) • Pumpkin • Red peppers • Sweet potatoes	900 mcg**
Vitamin B6	• Immune function • Nervous system function • Protein, carbohydrate, and fat metabolism • Red blood cell formation	• Chickpeas • Fruits (other than citrus) • Potatoes • Salmon • Tuna	1.7 mg
Vitamin B12	• Conversion of food into energy • Nervous system function • Red blood cell formation	• Dairy products • Eggs • Fortified cereals • Meat • Poultry • Seafood (e.g., clams, trout, salmon, haddock, tuna)	2.4 mcg
Vitamin C	• Antioxidant • Collagen and connective tissue formation Immune function • Wound healing	• Fruit (e.g., cantaloupe, citrus fruits, kiwifruit, and strawberries) • Juices (e.g., oranges, grapefruit, and tomato) • Vegetables (e.g., broccoli, Brussels sprouts, peppers, and tomatoes)	90 mg
Vitamin D (Nutrient to get more of)	• Blood pressure regulation • Bone growth • Calcium balance • Hormone production • Immune function • Nervous system function	• Beef liver • Egg yolks • Fish (e.g., flounder, herring, salmon, trout, and tuna) • Fish oil and cod liver oil • Fortified dairy products • Fortified orange juice • Fortified soy beverages • Fortified ready-to-eat cereals • Mushrooms	20 mcg**

VITAMIN	FUNCTION	SOURCES	DAILY VALUE
Vitamin E	• Antioxidant • Formation of blood vessels • Immune function	• Fortified cereals and juices • Green vegetables (e.g., spinach and broccoli) • Nuts and seeds • Peanuts and peanut butter • Vegetable oils	15 mg**
Vitamin K	• Blood clotting • Strong bones	• Green vegetables (e.g., broccoli, kale, spinach, turnip greens, collard greens, Swiss chard, mustard greens)	120 mcg

* The Daily Values are reference amounts of nutrients to consume or not to exceed each day.

— TABLE 17.3 —
MINERAL FUNCTIONS, SOURCES, AND DAILY NEEDS (VALUE)[71]

MINERAL	FUNCTION	SOURCES	DAILY VALUE*
Calcium (Nutrient to get more of)	• Blood clotting • Bone and teeth formation • Constriction and relaxation of blood vessels • Hormone secretion • Muscle contraction • Nervous system function	• Canned seafood with bones (e.g., salmon and sardines) • Dairy products • Fortified orange juice • Fortified soy beverages • Fortified ready-to-eat cereals • Green vegetables (e.g., kale, broccoli, and collard greens) • Tofu (made with calcium sulfate)	1,300 mg
Chloride	• Acid-base balance • Conversion of food into energy • Digestion • Fluid balance • Nervous system function	• Olives • Rye • Salt substitutes • Seaweeds (e.g., dulse and kelp) • Table salt and sea salt • Vegetables (e.g., celery, lettuce, and tomatoes)	2,300 mg
Chromium	• Insulin function • Protein, carbohydrate, and fat metabolism	• Broccoli • Fruits (e.g., apples and bananas) • Juices (e.g., grape and orange) • Meat • Spices (e.g., garlic and basil) • Turkey • Whole grains	35 mcg

MINERAL	FUNCTION	SOURCES	DAILY VALUE*
Copper	• Antioxidant • Bone formation • Collagen and connective tissue formation • Energy production • Iron metabolism • Nervous system function	• Chocolate and cocoa • Crustaceans and shellfish • Lentils • Nuts and seeds • Organ meats (e.g., liver) • Whole grains	0.9 mg
Iodine	• Growth and development • Metabolism • Reproduction • Thyroid hormone production	• Breads and cereals • Dairy products • Iodized salt • Potatoes • Seafood • Seaweed • Turkey	150 mcg
Iron (Nutrient to get more of)	• Energy production • Growth and development • Immune function • Red blood cell formation • Reproduction • Wound healing	• Beans, peas, and lentils • Eggs • Fruits (e.g., raisins and cantaloupe) • Green vegetables (e.g., asparagus, beet greens, broccoli, spinach, and swiss chard) • Meat • Nuts • Organ meats (e.g., liver) • Poultry • Seafood (e.g., crab, clams, sardines, shrimp, and oysters) • Seeds • Soy products (e.g., tofu) • Whole grain, enriched, and fortified breads, cereals, pasta, and rice	18 mg
Magnesium	• Blood pressure regulation • Blood sugar regulation • Bone formation • Energy production • Hormone secretion • Immune function • Muscle contraction • Nervous system function • Normal heart rhythm • Protein formation	• Avocados • Beans and peas • Dairy products • Fruits (e.g., bananas and raisins) • Green leafy vegetables (e.g., spinach) • Nuts and pumpkin seeds • Potatoes • Whole grains	420 mg

MINERAL	FUNCTION	SOURCES	DAILY VALUE*
Manganese	• Carbohydrate, protein, and cholesterol metabolism • Cartilage and bone formation • Wound healing	• Carbohydrate, protein, and cholesterol metabolism • Cartilage and bone formation • Wound healing	2.3 mg
Molybdenum	• Enzyme production	• Beans and peas • Nuts • Whole grains	45 mcg
Phosphorus	• Acid-base balance • Bone formation • Energy production and storage • Hormone activation	• Beans and peas • Dairy products • Meat • Nuts and seeds • Poultry • Seafood • Whole grain, enriched, and fortified cereals and breads	1,250 mg
Potassium (Nutrient to get more of)	• Blood pressure regulation • Carbohydrate metabolism • Fluid balance • Growth and development • Heart function • Muscle contraction • Nervous system function • Protein formation	• Beans • Dairy products (e.g., milk and yogurt) • Fruits (e.g., apricots, bananas, kiwifruit, cantaloupe, and grapefruit) • Juices (e.g., carrot and other vegetables juices, orange, pomegranate, and prune) • Seafood (e.g., clams, pollock, and trout) • Tomato products • Vegetables (e.g., potatoes, sweet potatoes, beet greens, and spinach)	4,700 mg
Selenium	• Antioxidant • Immune function • Reproduction • Thyroid function	• Eggs • Enriched pasta and rice • Meat • Nuts (e.g., Brazil nuts) and seeds • Poultry • Seafood • Whole grains	55 mcg

MINERAL	FUNCTION	SOURCES	DAILY VALUE*
Sodium (Nutrient to get less of)	• Acid-base balance • Blood pressure regulation • Fluid balance • Muscle contraction • Nervous system function	• Deli meat sandwiches • Pizza • Burritos and tacos • Soups • Savory snacks (e.g., chips, crackers, popcorn) • Poultry • Pasta mixed dishes • Burgers Egg dishes and omelets	2,300 mg
Zinc	• Growth and development • Immune function • Nervous system function • Protein formation • Reproduction • Taste and smell • Wound healing	• Beans and peas • Beef • Dairy products • Fortified cereals • Nuts • Poultry • Shellfish • Whole grains	11 mg

* The Daily Values are reference amounts of nutrients to consume or not to exceed each day.

Now that we've covered the macronutrients (carbohydrates, fats, and proteins) and micronutrients (vitamins, minerals, and phytonutrients). Let's tackle some other questions I often get from my clients and students.

CHAPTER 18

NUTRITION QUESTIONS ANSWERED

What Are Genetically Modified Organisms (GMOs)?

If a plant breed has a disease, there is sometimes a way to change its DNA to get rid of the disease. In other words, the plant becomes resistant to that disease. This is the idea behind genetically modified organisms. The DNA of our fruits and vegetables is sometimes changed so that it can survive attacks from certain diseases, insects, and other pests.

This is different from the cross-pollination experiments you may have learned about in elementary school, where pollen from one plant with a specific characteristic (color, for example) is transferred to the stigma of another plant with a different characteristic (a different color, in this case) to obtain a different result. The DNA is not changed in that case.

If you want to get technical, "The National Bioengineered Food Disclosure Standard defines bioengineered foods as those that contain detectable genetic material that has been modified through certain lab techniques and cannot be created through conventional breeding or found in nature."[72]

Are GMOs Safe?

GMOs are like any other food innovation. There is not enough evidence to conclude their health benefits or harms. Most dietitians I know feel that they cannot responsibly promote the safety of GMOs until they have this evidence. For this reason, stay away if you can.

Some anecdotal evidence suggests that eliminating GMOs can help with allergies and improve other health conditions. If you have a health condition, it might be worth trying to eliminate GMOs to see if the health condition improves. It certainly would not hurt.

What Foods Contain GMOs?

Organic food items are not genetically modified, and this may come as a surprise, but most produce is not genetically modified. However, there are some produce items that, if they are not organic, are more likely than not to be genetically modified. They are:

- Corn
- Soybeans
- Potatoes
- Papayas and
- Summer squash

> Read the ingredients list on the label to see if your food has any form of corn (including high fructose corn syrup) or soybeans. If it is not organic, it will almost always have GMOs.

GMOs seem to be everywhere because some genetically modified produce items are used to make things like cornstarch, corn oil, soybean oil, granulated sugar, corn syrup, and more.[73] These products are, in turn, used to make multiple processed foods. High fructose corn syrup, for example, is found in everything from:

- Sodas
- Ketchup

- BBQ sauce
- Applesauce
- Cereals
- Candy and candy bars
- Fake honey
- Ice cream
- Bread
- Yogurt and the list goes on

> Organic produce and organic processed foods contain fewer pesticides and no GMOs. If you can fit it into your budget, go for the organic.

The USDA publishes a list of bioengineered foods on its website.[74] This list includes the following foods:
- Alfalfa
- Apple (Golden Delicious, Granny Smith and Fuji varieties only)
- Canola
- Corn
- Cotton
- Eggplant (BARI Bt Begun varieties)
- Papaya (ringspot virus-resistant varieties)
- Pineapple (pink flesh varieties)
- Potato
- Salmon (AquAdvantage®)
- Soybean
- Squash (summer, coat protein-mediated virus-resistant varieties)
- Sugar beet
- Sugarcane (Bt insect-resistant varieties)

You don't have to worry about other fruits and vegetables being genetically modified. You can also look for the "Non GMO Project" stamp. But remember, because there is no stamp, that does not mean that it is genetically modified. Look for the ingredients listed above to avoid GMOs.

On Sodium, Salt, and Salt Alternatives

Sodium is a very important mineral necessary for life. It moderates our blood pressure, allows us to contract our muscles, and helps keep our cells healthy. Too much sodium can elevate blood pressure, which can lead to heart attacks and strokes, especially when combined with high saturated fat intake and stress.

An estimated 70% of our sodium intake comes from packaged or prepared foods.[75] That's right, that extra salt you may add to your dine-in/take-out meal or frozen dinner is only a small fraction of the salt already in your food. Just by preparing food at home, you can reduce your sodium intake significantly.

How Much Sodium Per Day?

It is recommended that the average American limit their sodium intake to less than 2,400 mg of sodium per day. Check out the sodium levels of certain common fast foods in Table 18.1. These foods do not include extra fixings like double burgers with bacon and extra cheese, supersizing of the French fries, or meat lover's pizza, just the basics. I have seen some burgers with 3,200 milligrams of sodium (which is 140% of the percent daily value).

— TABLE 18.1 —
SODIUM IN POPULAR FAST-FOODS

FOOD	SODIUM (MILLIGRAMS)	% DAILY VALUE
1 Fast food burger with cheese	1100	50%
1 Medium French fry	250	10%
1 Medium milkshake	250	10%
1 Small cheese and pepperoni pizza slice	400	17%
1 Beef taco	500	22%
1 Small ham and cheese sub	800	35%
1 Chicken alfredo dinner	2200	92%

One creamy pasta dish can easily have nearly 100% or more of the 2,400 mg of sodium recommended daily. Eating more than this will bring us above the sodium amount our body needs. I must again emphasize that the point of sharing this is not to make you go crazy about crunching numbers, but instead, it is to create awareness. If a plain cheeseburger has 50% of the sodium for the day, how much would a double cheeseburger with bacon have? What about a super-sized fry instead of a medium fry? What if you add garlic bread to that chicken alfredo dinner? It all adds up.

Regarding packaged foods, potato chips, canned soups, and salty crackers are not the only high-sodium foods. Table 18.2 has the sodium content of certain foods you may not expect to have high sodium levels. Read those labels, and don't forget to pay attention to the portion size.

— TABLE 18.2 —
SODIUM IN UNSUSPECTING PROCESSED FOODS

FOOD	SODIUM (MILLIGRAMS)	% DAILY VALUE
Bread (2 slices)	250	10%
Sweetened cereals (2/3 cup)	200	8%
Ketchup (1 tablespoon)	180	8%
Hot sauce (1 teaspoon)	200	8%
Ranch dressing (1 tablespoon)	150	6%

You can check the restaurant website for information on sodium for a large chain restaurant meal. If you ask, they might even have the information available at the restaurant. The smaller restaurants more than likely will not have this information. In those cases, you would have to make estimations based on what you know about similar foods at other restaurants.

> Sodium can sneak up in foods you would least expect. Two slices of bread can have 250 mg of sodium, cereals can have 200 mg per serving, and one tablespoon of ketchup can have almost 200 mg of sodium. Pay attention!

Salt vs. Sodium

Salt contains sodium, but it is not sodium. Salt has a sodium chloride structure and forms the crystals we are all familiar with. Sodium is a stand-alone element that can also be found in food naturally.

Celery has a salty taste and is a great vegetable for flavoring soups and other dishes because it contains sodium. It has 80 milligrams of sodium, about 3% of the %DV. Table 18.3 has some other natural sources of sodium and their sodium quantities.

— TABLE 18.3 —
SODIUM IN POPULAR VEGETABLES

FOOD	SODIUM (MILLIGRAMS)	% DAILY VALUE
Celery (2 stalks)	80	3%
Carrots (2 medium)	70	3%
Broccoli (1 cup)	40	2%
Brussels Sprouts (1 cup)	25	1%
Collard Greens (½ cup)	20	1%

Eating foods that naturally contain sodium provides us with the sodium we need. It even leaves room for seasoning with salt without taking us over the top.

Are Some Salts Healthier Than Others?

Most salts on the market have sodium, so whatever you decide to use, it is still important not to overdo it. To make it simple, there are two main types of salt: refined and unrefined.

- ☑ **Refined Salt** is processed salt that has been stripped of many of its nutrients, like refined carbohydrates, oils, etc. However, a very important nutrient, iodine, has been added to refined salt as a public health response to an iodine deficiency problem in the United States.

    Iodine is necessary for healthy thyroid function, hormone regulation, and metabolism. Adding iodine to salt (also known as iodized salt) has helped many to avoid problems like hypothyroidism and hyperthyroidism.

☑ **Unrefined salt** is unprocessed salt with most of its original nutrients. Himalayan and Celtic salts, for example, have calcium, magnesium, iron, zinc, potassium, and several other nutrients you won't find in refined salt. So, we get an extra nutrition boost when we use Himalayan, Celtic, or other unrefined salts.

> Unrefined salts like Himalayan Sea Salts have more nutrients than refined salts, but they cost more. If it is not in your budget to purchase the more expensive salts, you can get your nutrition from other sources.

Unrefined salt may have a stronger flavor than refined salt, so you are less likely to use it as much. I recommend unrefined salts if they fit your budget. However, there is no need to worry if it does not.

What About Salt Alternatives?

The best way to reduce sodium intake is to eat homemade foods in place of processed and prepared foods. Another way to reduce sodium is to use a salt alternative. I typically recommend salt alternatives to individuals who have certain health conditions. The Mrs. Dash line of seasoning is a popular alternative to salt. I like it because it is a natural blend of naturally nutrient-rich herbs and spices that many of my students and clients like to use.

On Weight Management

Weight management is one of the most popular topics that I receive questions about. First, allow me to encourage you to love yourself where you are, no matter how big or how small. Second, please know that if you decide to lose weight, that does not mean that you do not love yourself. Third, when approaching weight management, consider focusing on health instead of weight; it is often a more productive and sustainable strategy.

Focusing on health means being aware of what we put in our bodies and why we put it there. Are you eating more than your body needs, or are you not eating enough of what your body needs? If so, why or why not? Digging into that very question is very powerful. The paragraphs that follow will help us get into what and why.

Weight Management: What Are You Eating?

Per Chapter 12, when someone comes to me for weight management advice, the first thing I do is a food recall for a typical weekday and weekend day if they are different. I will add up the approximate number of calories and nutrients that the person is taking in and make comparisons to their actual needs based on a number of factors.

When I show my clients the difference in the numbers, they are typically blown away. They often don't realize how few calories they need versus how much they take in. They also don't realize gaps in their nutrient intake. For example, they may not be getting enough fiber or iron, or whatever it may be. After identifying that, we fill in the gaps.

This is a helpful exercise, but a less labor-intensive way to fill in those gaps is to make sure we are eating lots of different colored fruits, vegetables, and other plant-based whole foods mentioned throughout this book.

Weight Management: Why Are You Eating It?

Another important factor to consider when it comes to weight management is the impact of stress on our food choices and how our bodies process food. It is much greater than you might think.

I often hear people say, *"I just need to eat less/more, and I will be fine."* While that may be true, one reason you might be eating the quantities and types of food you eat may be stress. If that is the case and you don't recognize it as a factor, that can affect your ability to reach your weight/health goal. This is why stress management is important.

Chapters 19 and 20 dive more into stress management and how loving on yourself and giving yourself grace is a form of stress management. When you love yourself, you recognize your God-given right to rest and take time out of your day to take care of yourself. I bet that if you sit down and think about all of your many responsibilities, you can find a window for yourself. If you can't find a window for yourself, pray/meditate about it—your answer will come. Sometimes, it helps to talk it out with others too.

Giving yourself a window that will allow you to de-stress and love yourself will spill over into other decisions that you make for yourself. Including the food that you eat.

Even with that, you will not always do the best thing for yourself—that is where giving yourself grace comes in. It truly is ok if you don't make the best choices. You'll do better tomorrow. Move on. Just remember to go back to loving yourself, and when you forget to create that window, go back to the prayer/meditation closet and find it.

Weight Management: Exercise

Exercise is important for health and weight maintenance but may not be as useful for weight loss/gain as you might think. In fact, health professionals in my circle say that weight management is 80% diet and 20% exercise. I would argue that it is 50% stress management/wellness, 40% diet and 10% exercise.

Before elaborating on this point, I want to emphasize that exercise is one of the most important things you can do for your health. While it is important for weight maintenance, it also boosts the immune system, regulates blood sugar, improves mood, provides energy, prevents arthritic pain, relieves stress, helps with sleep, speeds up your metabolism, and so much more. So please, exercise.

I bring up this point because often, people will exercise for an hour at the gym, only to come out and get a caramel macchiato, some other sugary beverage, or a protein bar. A typical 16-ounce café drink or soda/lemonade is going to run you 200 calories. Depending on your workout, you may have burned 100–300 calories. So, many of the calories you just burned off, you just added back.

You still are going to get all of the other benefits of the exercise mentioned earlier. And the metabolism boost is going to help you burn those calories a little bit easier so whether you drink it or not, it's a fantastic thing for your health. However, it is hard to out-exercise a diet with significantly more calories than we need.

Another thing that can help with weight management is portion control. Let's get into it.

Weight Management: Portion Control (It is Budget Friendly!)

A common recommendation for weight management is portion control. This book presents several reasons not to obsess about counting calories. By focusing on plant-based whole foods, there is no need to calorie count. However, if we are eating processed and prepared foods, there is something to be said about sticking to the recommended serving size listed on the nutrition facts labels. Not only does it save calories, but it saves money. A cereal box can last two or three times as long just by following the recommended serving size. Pouring cereal into a bowl without knowing the serving size can cause one to eat three or more servings. There is no harm in using a measuring cup or measuring spoon for your servings. Consider that as another way to save.

On Chewing Your Food Well

When you get a chance, pay attention to how fast you eat. Do you take two bites, swallow, and then you are on to the next bite? Or do you chew your food until it is in small pieces and then swallow?

I ask because digestion begins in the mouth. You have an enzyme called salivary amylase in your saliva that breaks down carbohydrates in the food and makes digestion easier. When we chew our food into little pieces, we allow that amylase to do its job right, making digestive problems less likely.

Also, our bodies have something called a satiety signal. That is the signal our brains give us to let us know that we have eaten enough. It takes about 20 minutes for that signal to take effect after we begin eating. If we eat our entire plate within a five-to-ten-minute timespan, we will not receive that satiety signal in that timeframe and will want to keep eating.

When we take our time and chew our food until the food is in small pieces, not only do we digest our food better, but we give ourselves time to receive the satiety signal.

Consider being conscious of how fast you eat and making a concerted effort to chew your food well if you are not doing so already.

* * *

You are now armed with information that will help you improve your health through food. In the next section, we will investigate how we can improve our health through stress management and wellness.

PART 3
THE WORK

TAKING CARE OF YOU

CHAPTER 19

RELAX AND GIVE YOURSELF A BREAK

Choosing to eat a nutritious diet can be difficult. We are all familiar with the cycle. We try to eat right, we fail, then stress ourselves out because we failed, and then we stress ourselves out about trying it one more time. Only this time, we want to try something different, but this time, we have to figure out what we are going to try. We finally find a new guru/diet to follow, we fail, and the cycle continues. It adds layers upon layers of stress to many of our already very stressful lives. This chapter is all about getting rid of the stress associated with that cycle because nobody has time for that!

To eliminate some of that stress, it is helpful to know where to find and prepare healthy foods that fit our budgets as we did in parts one and two. But let's talk about the elephant in the room: What is the cause of these difficulties in choosing healthy foods? Here are a few:

1. Unhealthy and ultra-processed food marketing (often beginning with marketing to children, which follows them through life)
2. Easy access to these ultra-processed foods
3. Food addictions, often aided by numbers 1 and 2
4. Taste preferences (often informed by numbers 1, 2, and 3)

  a. In one of the nutrition classes I used to teach, I had a picture of a hamburger and French fries and a picture of a piece of salmon with roasted potatoes and asparagus (or some version of that). I asked the class which one they would choose if they had a choice between the two and did not have to pay for either one? Most everyone, teenagers and adults alike, said they would choose the hamburger and fries.
5. Emotions
  a. If you are like me, you eat a lot when you are happy/excited, eat junk when you are sad/depressed, and if you are stressed, you barely eat at all. Of course, everyone is different, but how we feel emotionally often influences what we decide we are going to eat.
6. Stress
  a. When you have a million worries on your mind and a million things to do, you want something quick and convenient that suits your tastes. Numbers 1, 2, and 3 then take over.

Let's Talk About Stress

Stress is our body's physical and mental reactions to environmental changes. Our bodies are designed to handle all kinds of stress, whether positive, negative, short-term, or long-term. The best scenario for the body is positive, long-term stress with short-term moments of negative stress. Our body is designed to deal with negative stress. Some might even argue that certain types of negative stress are good. When the negative stress is constant, however, problems arise.

Many of us experience negative, long-term stress with short-term/long-term moments of positive stress without even knowing it.

This chapter will help you identify the negative and positive stressors that you can do something about.

This chapter will also help you to work on achieving positive long-term stress with short-term moments of negative stress, or what I am going to call the *net-positive stress zone*, at no financial cost. Before doing that, I'd like to remind you to take things step by step. Start with what works for you and build from there. But first, a little bit of biochemistry.

Hormones

Hormones play an important role in every aspect of our health. Let's consider the hormone insulin as an example of how hormones work.

1. When glucose (sugar) from the carbohydrates that we eat enters the bloodstream, the sugar tells the pancreas to release insulin.
2. The pancreas releases insulin which picks up the sugar floating around in the blood.
3. The insulin carries the sugar to the cells.
4. As mentioned in Chapter 14, the cells allow the sugar in and convert it to energy.
5. This energy is then used to activate different reactions in the body that are responsible for everything from moving to thinking and breathing.

This is just one of the untold numbers of hormonal systems that are activated in response to the food that we eat.

Stress Hormones

Just like food activates multiple hormonal systems, stress does too. Your brain detects stressful (positive or negative) situations and releases specific hormones (called stress hormones) that activate multiple hormone systems. There are multiple sources of positive and negative stressors that can activate these stress hormones.

Positive Forms of Stress

1. Physical stress (from exercise/sports, roller coaster rides, deep breathing, etc.)
2. Mental stress (from peace of mind, safety, new home, new/stable job, etc.)
3. Emotional stress (from relationships, good news in the media, etc.)
4. Spiritual stress (from a good sermon, spiritual song, prayer, meditation, etc.)

Negative Forms of Stress

1. Physical stress (from accidents, health problems, busy schedules/time constraints, etc.)
2. Mental stress (from worry, anxiety, unsafe environments, imposter syndrome, etc.)
3. Emotional stress (from relationships, loss of a loved one, bad news in the media, etc.)
4. Spiritual stress (from feeling like you're not fulfilling your purpose, etc.)

When the stress from positive sources outweighs the stress from negative sources, we have net-positive stress. **Stress management** is the effort one makes to achieve net-positive stress levels.

Stress Impacts the Way We Digest Food

The types of food that we eat are not the only things that impact digestion. You may have heard of the stress hormone cortisol. Constant distressful events, negative thoughts, unsafe environments, etc., can cause cortisol to float around at high levels in the blood, eventually impacting the way we digest food.

One study found that "chronically elevated cortisol may lead to impaired digestive function—e.g., increased intestinal permeability, impaired absorption of micronutrients, abdominal pain or discomfort, and local and systemic inflammation."[76]

> This chapter is about achieving positive, long-term stress with short term moments of negative stress. What I am going to call net-positive stress.

This is why when people ask me what they should do to manage their weight, blood pressure, and other diet-related issues, one of my first questions is, "What are you doing to manage your stress?" I know they are looking for food solutions, but because stress impacts us in so many ways, to not address it would be missing the forest for the trees.

Stress does not only impact our health biochemically via digestion, but also, it impacts our health, behaviorally via our food choices.

Stress Affects Our Choices (Good and Bad)

Chances are, if I am experiencing net-negative stress, I am less likely to think about what I am going to eat. I will just eat what I know will satisfy my hunger and help bring me comfort.

Chances are that if I am experiencing net-positive stress levels, I will have more mental capacity to do things a bit differently when it comes to food. It could be something as simple as planning to bring a piece of fruit to work to snack on instead of eating the little chocolates available in the break room.

Stress hormones activate a system different from, yet equally complicated as, the hormone insulin. Eventually, this complicated process can affect the part of our brain responsible for decision-making, problem-solving, and organization (the prefrontal cortex).[77] So not only do we have stress itself impacting our life/food choices and how we digest food, but this stress is aided and abetted by a transformational change in our brain that impacts our choices.

Achieving Net-Positive Stress Levels

Stress management is not important just so that we can make healthier food choices but also so that we can experience life in a more peaceful, fulfilling, and even pain-free way. In my years of counseling patients, including those with cancer, it was amazing how something as simple as deep breathing or going on a walk would help alleviate some of their anxieties and even help relieve some of their physical symptoms. There are several stress management techniques that cost us absolutely nothing financially (except maybe a journal, which is not necessary, but recommended). I'd like to walk you through some of them. But first, I'd like to ask you like I ask my clients…

> **What do you do to reduce stress in your life right now?**

Have you ever asked yourself this question? Think about that question. What do you come up with? If you got nothin', that's ok; that's what this chapter is for. If you have something, write it down here or in a journal.

_____

_____

_____

I mentioned earlier that nutrition/diet is often taught in isolation. We talk about vitamins, minerals, proteins, and food groups, but we often don't discuss the stressors and environments impacting our food decisions. We focus on diet trends, factory-made alternatives (like artificial sweeteners), individual foods/nutrients, and individual studies that confuse us with each reporting of the findings.

Sometimes, going beyond nutrition means a little bit of work is involved, and I included exercises in the following sections to aid you in doing that work. These exercises will help you identify some stressors that may impact your food choices (and other life choices). After identifying those stressors, we will move on to managing the stress that comes along with those stressors. Let's get started with exercise 1.

> We cannot control everything that happens in our lives, but we can manage how we deal with what happens.

Exercise 1: Stop to think for a moment about what you consider when purchasing a particular food and write it down here or in your journal.

1. _____
2. _____
3. _____
4. _____
5. _____

Now, if you've ever decided to change your diet in any way (it could be a fad diet or just a desire to eat more vegetables), write down the other factors you considered when purchasing a particular food.

1. _____
2. _____
3. _____
4. _____
5. _____

* * *

This exercise helps us understand what drives our seemingly simple decisions and gives us a better sense of the mental hoops we deal with every day. Our focus is on food choices, but this exercise can be applied to life choices in general. The exercise also puts us on a path to doing something about all those layers of stuff that we often don't address.

> Sit Down
> Become Aware
> Problem-Solve

Trying to understand the mental hoops may seem like another layer we have to deal with, but this is a classic "an ounce of prevention is worth a pound of cure" situation. Taking minutes out of your week, or month even, to sit down, become aware, and problem-solve can help to reduce or eliminate some of the other layers of stress we may be dealing with. This will move us closer to the net-positive stress zone.

One thing I noticed in my personal life and over the course of my career working with so many different people is that many of us don't problem-solve. We assume that there is nothing we can do about our stressors, and we just let them pile on. When often, there is something we can do.

Some of your stressors may have been exposed in exercise 1. Perhaps you notice that you bring home certain foods that you may not want to because your family complains if you don't. If so, what are some things that you can do about that? Perhaps a conversation with your family about the importance of health and making small changes will help. What about setting small health goals together? Perhaps, trying new things periodically will help.

Perhaps you are a single parent and don't have time to think about what you are going to give your family, so you go with what is familiar even though you know it is not healthy. Is there someone you can ask to help you with some of your responsibilities so you can find time? Is there a family member, a neighbor, or a member of your religious community that you trust? A coworker who you've worked with and trust.

Even your children can help out. It can be something as little as folding clothes, helping with dinner, making their own bed, cleaning their own room, or cleaning another room in the house. The more we engage children in these types of activities, the more responsibility they learn. And the earlier we engage them, the better. Four-year-olds can do a lot more than you might think. Doing "activities" is great for your children.

This first stress management technique is all about asking for help as a way to manage stress and problem-solve.

Stress Management Technique #1: Ask for Help

You would be surprised by the number of people who would be willing to help you. It could be a family member, a friend, a coworker, a boss, a human resource department, a fellow believer, a religious leader, an organization, or a business. Asking for help is so powerful yet so underutilized. Taking all of this into consideration, complete exercise 2 below.

Exercise 2: Stressors and problem-solving

WHAT ARE THREE (3) STRESSORS IN MY LIFE?	WHAT CAN I DO TO REMOVE SOME OF THE STRESS ASSOCIATED WITH THIS STRESSOR?	WHO CAN I ASK FOR HELP? AND WHAT CAN I ASK THEM TO DO?
1.		
2.		
3.		

Writing it down is the first step. The next step is building up the courage to ask. "Ye have not, because ye ask not" was a scripture my former fellow church folks and family quoted often. "Pride cometh before the fall" was another one. Taken out of context as they may be in this situation, they help to explain why some of our needs go unmet (i.e., you didn't ask) and what happens when we don't ask because of our pride (we become stressed out even more).

There are a lot of kind people out there who are willing to help and won't judge you. More than you might think. And if you do happen to come across that judgy, mean person who is looking for something in return, be grateful that their true character has been revealed to you and move on. At the end of the day, who cares what they think? I mean, really—who cares?

We live so much of our lives worried about what others think, and I get it, we all have a need to be accepted. Even as I write this book, I am thinking about getting acceptance. But it comes to a point that if I look for acceptance from everyone, I am never going to put anything out there. People are going to criticize and judge us no matter what we do, and if we don't take risks because of fear, we won't get any help or do anything.

Now, the next sentence is something you might have to brace for, so prepare yourself for a reality check. Sometimes we have these fears of others because we are the judgy, mean ones looking for something in return (Ask me how I know.). I mean, yes, we see others be judgy and mean on TV in the media and even in our personal lives, and that makes us leery of everybody. But often, it's not what we see in the media that makes us leery; it's that we see ourselves in others, and we don't trust people because that is the way we are (Again, ask me how I know.).

It is worth exploring if you suspect that that may be you. Not so that you can beat yourself up about it but so that you can become better. Life is about becoming better constantly, for ourselves, first and foremost, and for others. The better we are to ourselves, the more capacity we have to help others, and then the more capacity others have to help us. It is a beautiful cycle.

Asking for help does not mean asking anybody for anything and everything; just use discretion. Some people you already know not to trust because they showed you who they are. But some people showed you that you can trust them, and you still don't trust them because you don't trust anybody. Sometimes you might be wrong, but I think you will be pleasantly surprised by how beautiful people really are. And if they say no, that is not rejection; they just may not have the capacity.

Asking for help builds relationships (something else that helps with stress) while lifting a heavy weight. It is often also beneficial to the person you ask. This brings us to our next stress management technique.

Stress Management Technique #2: Social Support and Building Relationships

The Blue Zones book by Dan Buettner highlights seven communities in the world with a relatively high rate of individuals over the age of 100 years. One of the commonalities of all seven communities, despite being in totally different parts of the world, is that they all had strong social networks.

Social support could be a strong family unit, religious or friend group, support network, book club, painting/cooking/gardening/sewing group, contractors sharing ideas group, volunteer group, sports team (pickleball is a great social sport), or any group where you share common interests and support each other.

In a world that is becoming less and less social due to social media and working from home, it seems like it's harder to build relationships than it was years ago. And listen, I know that being part of social groups eventually means that you are going to have to deal with the shenanigans because, let's face it, folks will be folks. I see you, and I hear you. However, brace yourself for another reality check. Sometimes, we are those folks creating the shenanigans, and we don't know it. Again, ask me how I know.

It is hard to do a self-check, painful even, but it's necessary for personal growth. I am convinced that if we all did self-checks, there would be a lot less shenanigans we would have to deal with. I mean, everything can't always be everybody else's fault. This does not mean we take the blame for everything. Instead, it means that we acknowledge that sometimes we may play a role.

I remember going to therapy with my husband. I went into therapy thinking he had all the issues and that he was the problem. On the first meeting, our therapist took a good look at me and said, "You need to see me individually." I was shocked, in disbelief even. However, I did individual counseling despite my disbelief, and he helped me to see where I was the problem and how I wasn't the angel that I thought I was. My husband had things to work on, too, but because we both took stock of our stuff (and boy, was there stuff), we were able to navigate many of the challenges of our marriage and are constantly building our relationship by working on ourselves. If you are in a relationship with someone who is not willing to work on themselves, that presents another problem that is unhealthy for you. Consider talking to someone you trust about this.

Therapy is very helpful, but if you don't have the time and money right now, you can do some internal reflection. It can start with recognizing that you can be wrong sometimes, but know that it is ok to be wrong, especially because we can always course correct. Some people might try to define you based on a mistake that you made or a character flaw you might have. Remember that your mistakes and flaws don't define your being; they are more like wounds that need healing, not the entire body itself.

One book that helped me with this is The Four Agreements book by Don Miguel Ruiz. It is a book of Toltec wisdom. One of the four agreements is: "Don't Take Anything Personal." The things people say about you are just that, the things *people* say about you. Don't take any of it personally, *positive* or negative. Once you start to believe other peoples' thoughts about you, you form an agreement that has nothing to do with the real you. Then we start living our entire lives based on what *they* said about us. I'd like to put some emphasis on how even the positive things should not be taken personally.

I grew up being admired for being a goody-two-shoes Christian. Which basically meant that I didn't smoke, cuss, have sex (outside of marriage), do drugs, or drink. Oh yeah, and I got good grades in school, volunteered, sang in the choir and I could pray a mean prayer. All of the positive reinforcements made me feel like I was on the right track and was living my life the way it was supposed to be lived. Only to realize later that I was judgy, even mean sometimes, and that I was/am (Give me a break, I am working on it.) selfish. I also realized that I was living my life in a way that was pleasing to the people around me (All of the positive reinforcement made me feel good about it.) but not necessarily pleasing to the creator and what I was created to be.

The stress relief that comes along with living your truth and not taking what others say about you personally is immeasurable and helps move us closer to a net-positive stress level.

Allow me to also mention that getting to a place of healing those wounds (that don't make up our entire being--you gotta remember that) means healing from trauma and other things we may have experienced in our lives that we've never dealt with. Yeah, I know it can get ugly, and diving deeper into it goes beyond the scope of this book. But know that awareness is the first step. Doing work to heal these wounds will better equip you to have healthy relationships and having healthy relationships and social networks (the key word is healthy) is a powerful way to manage stress and optimize our health. As we've seen with the Blue Zones.

So as not to become too overwhelmed, take things step by step, even if it is starting with a simple question in the morning, "How can I heal (or become better) today?" I've learned that the act of asking the question AND waiting/looking for the answer will yield results specific to you and your situation.

Another simple yet powerful question I ask in the morning is, "Dear God, what am I supposed to learn today?" I try to leave myself open to things I need to learn about myself (good and bad), others, and the world around me. The life lessons are there for us to learn and sometimes we can't move on to the next phase in our lives until we learn those lessons. If you feel stuck in your life, what is the lesson that God/the universe is trying to teach you that you are not paying him/it any mind about? Seek out the lesson and course correct. Your life will change.

And finally, to not become too overwhelmed with all of this, it is important to give yourself grace constantly. This brings us to stress management technique #3.

(Please note that we are going to get to more traditional stress management techniques, but bear with me as we go through some unconventional ones that get to the root.)

Stress Management Technique #3: Give Yourself Grace

Oxford's definition of the word grace is "courteous, goodwill." Courteous means "polite, respectful, or considerate in manner." Goodwill means "friendly, helpful, or cooperative feelings or attitudes." Are you polite, respectful, and considerate to yourself? Are you friendly and helpful to yourself? Take a moment to reflect on how respectful and considerate you are to yourself.

Exercise 3: Write down the ways that you are respectful and considerate to yourself here or in your journal.

_____

_____

_____

Exercise 4: Write down the ways that you are not polite and respectful to yourself here or in your journal.

_____

_____

_____

While we embrace the idea that we can be wrong sometimes, sometimes, it has nothing to do with us and that is important to recognize also. Consider our food choices, for example. How often do we beat ourselves up because we ate the bacon double cheeseburger? Allow me to let you in on something that you probably already know: There are reckless, conspicuous, and inconspicuous individuals and groups that influence our food decisions and make it incredibly difficult for us to make healthy choices. You *cannot* be responsible for that recklessness so don't take that on as a fault of your own. Stop feeling guilty for that. Let that go! It's not in your control. What is in your control is how you navigate their shenanigans and how you treat yourself.

Even for the things that are in your control, stop feeling guilty for that too. Guilt is one of the least productive human emotions when it comes to our diets because it makes us feel bad about ourselves, which can lead to a desire for traditional comfort foods. That can lead to more guilt and a vicious cycle.

Being healthy does not only involve what you put into your body but also what you put into your mind. So what? You ate the hamburger, pizza, French fries, and milkshake in one sitting. Acknowledge that it wasn't the best choice for your health but move on.

You have more important things to tell yourself. Like, how wonderful you are. Like, how you made it this far because of how smart you are. Like, how kind you are to others and how the world is a better place because you are in it. Like, how your mistakes don't define you. Like, it's ok. Get used to giving yourself a break and speaking well of yourself no matter how you feel. You don't have to be perfect.

> Give yourself a break—several breaks, in fact. Show yourself kindness and speak lovingly to yourself about yourself.

I gave you some examples of what it sounds like to give yourself grace. Now stop and think about what giving yourself grace sounds like to you. What does it feel like to you? If the thought of showing yourself kindness, giving yourself a break, and speaking lovingly to yourself is tough, it just means that you haven't practiced doing it enough. Here is some practice.

Exercise 5: Put this book down, pause, and think about what it means to give yourself grace. After thinking about it, write down what you came up with here or in your journal.

_____

_____

_____

_____

Exercise 6: Now, practice giving yourself grace. Write down ways that you are going to practice giving yourself grace.

_____

_____

_____

_____

_____

Here are some more ways to give yourself grace:
- ☑ Pat yourself on the back.
- ☑ Tell yourself that what you did and what you ate yesterday is ok and that it's ok not to be perfect. Pat yourself on the back for acknowledging that.
- ☑ Look yourself in the mirror and tell yourself that you are strong, you are beautiful, you are kind, you are wise, you are encouraging, you take care of others, you beat cancer, whatever it is. Remind yourself.
- ☑ Pick out your favorite feature and tell yourself why it's your favorite feature. If you don't have a favorite feature, find one. It can be a physical trait, a personality trait, a spiritual trait, or an emotional trait. It could be something like: "I love that I speak up for myself at work." Or "I love that I controlled myself enough not to knock my coworker's head off when he/she was getting on my last nerve."
- ☑ Now, this might be a tough one for some of you, but look yourself in the mirror and say, "I love you," and mean it. If nobody else loves you, love yourself, flaws and all. Because you are more than your flaws. I don't care what anybody says about you. You are more than what others have reduced you to (or put you on a pedestal for).

Please note that giving yourself grace does not mean that you will escape consequences. If you commit a crime, you may have to go to jail. If you eat bad food regularly, you may get a diet-related disease. Giving yourself grace also is not an excuse to just love on yourself all day and become an egomaniac because it could indeed turn into that if we are not careful. Neither is it an excuse not to grow and make better decisions for yourself. It is quite the opposite.

Giving yourself grace means that you stop punishing yourself when you do something that is not in your best interest or the interest of others. It gives us the motivation to do the wiser thing next time. Beating ourselves up breeds hopelessness and discouragement. Grace removes the negative mental stress associated with beating ourselves up and can move us closer to the net-positive stress zone.

Since grace is so important, let's pencil it into our day.

Exercise 7: Choose one time during the day when you are going to give yourself grace. Put it on your calendar, set the timer—even if it's for one minute out of the day—and write that grace time (shall we call it?) below or in your journal.

Practice, Practice, Practice

Once you've chosen a time to give yourself grace, try to stick to it. Put up a reminder if you have to. This designated time is practice. As you stick with it, over time, you will start to give yourself grace throughout the day without having to schedule it. It will become part of how you think and a constant deposit in your positive stress bank.

> It's ok to not be perfect, it's ok to have flaws, it's ok. I'm not kidding. Remind yourself in the mirror—and say, "It's ok for me not to be perfect." Now give yourself a break!

Stress Management Technique #4: Release the Guilt

Much of the stress we experience around food is associated with the guilt we feel when we make unhealthy food choices. Do any of the following statements sound familiar to you?

"I shouldn't be eating that."

"I am going to pay for this later."

"You are such a loser; why do you keep eating that?"

"I know I shouldn't be giving this to my family, but…"

Those statements give fuel to guilt, and that guilt provides a breeding ground for more negative thoughts that lead to discouragement. Combine that with a low cash flow and a food industry that purposely promotes addictive and harmful foods, and you have another vicious cycle into the negative stress zone. Release that guilt and stop the cycle by giving yourself grace.

Fad and Prescriptive Diets Can Cause Guilt

Now that you are giving yourself grace and are releasing yourself from guilt; let's talk about dieting. Dieting involves depriving yourself of various foods or creating a food regimen that is often not biologically sustainable. Fad diets (to be distinguished from our definition of diet) create an environment of constant self-critique and punishment that eventually leads to self-defeat. Oftentimes, they are so extreme that they leave out essential nutrients and lead to health problems.

Instead of depriving yourself, the only thing I am going to recommend for you to do is

> **add new things to what you currently eat and listen to your body when it talks.**

There is no need to beat yourself up when you eat the donut or the extra piece of bread. It's ok. Next time, try to add the healthy stuff first. If you want to or need to eliminate certain ingredients from your diet, like sugar or gluten, that is fine. However, that can be a struggle for many. If that is your goal, a very effective and more permanent way to eliminate a particular food is to wean yourself off slowly like we did with the soda in Chapter 14.

When you continue adding new nutritious foods to your diet, you automatically stop eating some nutrient-empty foods without even realizing it. Many of the people that I work with feel that they don't have to deprive themselves because they find that their tastes have changed. They wind up not wanting many of the foods they ate before.

Release the guilt of eating unhealthy food, and give yourself grace. Now, let's talk about gratitude.

Stress Management Technique #5: Put Some Gratitude on It

We used to kid our parents because if we ever had a problem, it seemed like all they used to tell us to do was put some Vaseline on it. You got a bruise? Put some Vaseline on it. You broke a leg? Put some Vaseline on it? Do you have a headache? Put some Vaseline on it. Whatever it was, you just put Vaseline on it, and it would be better. To bring home the point of this section, I'd like to borrow that phrase and change out one word…

"Put some gratitude on it."

Although it didn't seem quite right to use Vaseline for everything, it seems to work for gratitude. No matter how hard things are, there always seems to be something to be grateful for. And searching for that thing to be grateful for, even in the hardest of times, seems to somehow make things seem better and reduce stress. Research even suggests that practicing gratitude may lower signs of heart disease and increase positive emotions.[78]

If you are not used to practicing gratitude, here is some gratitude practice for you.

Exercise 8: List one thing you are grateful for and write it below or in your journal.

_____

_____

You can plan it into your day, or you can do it when you get overwhelmed with thoughts and worries to help you calm down. While you are at it, take a few deep breaths (More on that later.). You will feel the stress relief and make another deposit into your positive stress zone.

Stress Management Technique #6: Speak Healing Words, Always

During my prayer time, amid a ton of frustration I was allowed to build up in me, I heard the words, "Speak healing words, always." These four words revolutionized my life.

I thought about what it means to speak healing words, and this is what came to mind. Speak in a way that will bring healing to yourself (most importantly), others, and society. Here are a few examples of healing words:

- ☑ I don't feel well today, but I will get better.
- ☑ His/her actions are not healthy for me, so I will heal from a distance so s/he cannot do it again. I hope and pray that s/he learns from his/her mistakes and does not do it to anyone else.
- ☑ I wholeheartedly disagree with that politician's actions, but I can still hope that something clicks with him/her and that from now on, s/he does the right thing for the people s/he is supposed to serve.

A far cry from the "she is an idiot" and "I can't stand him" that I was used to speaking. The concept is simple, if it doesn't bring healing, then don't speak it. In practice, however, it is a very difficult challenge. Especially for me because it made me aware of how often I don't speak healing words. I leaned more towards harmful words and didn't even know until that moment in my prayer time that I was challenged to always speak healing words.

I still catch myself not speaking healing words, but here is what I figured out; when I am on my rant or am getting myself worked up and speaking those harmful words, if I make a conscious effort to speak healing words, the more my thoughts change and the calmer I get. It's like an instant stress reliever, peace-of-mind giver even.

I was saying some cruel things about people who I felt wronged me. I was constantly angry and stressing myself out because I didn't know how to pay them back for the pain they inflicted on me. The moment I decided to heal and not be hurt by their actions was the moment I got free from the anger and desire to speak harmful words about them. I realized that those harmful words served only to make me more frustrated and angry. Unhinged anger is a giant unsung stressor on our bodies. Stressors can cause hormonal changes that translate to illness, including high blood pressure and obesity.[79]

I also noticed that some of my anger and the desire to speak ill of others came from jealousy. For some reason, I felt better when I was saying that a person "wasn't all that." When I started speaking healing words, I tried to look at the positive in those people instead of looking at the negative. Turns out, I feel even better when I can see the beauty in someone than I feel when I try to tear them down with my words because I am jealous.

Perhaps you grew up in an environment where gossip was the thing to do (most media and TV are basically gossip now), and now it is second nature to you. Perhaps you liked the attention you got from making jokes about others when you were a kid, and now that is your lifeblood. Perhaps, you had a difficult childhood and have legit reasons to be angry, but you never worked through those issues. It's ok to acknowledge the things that cause us to say words that are not so healing, whether it's anger, hurt, jealousy, habit, to get attention, or whatever. Now let's do something about it with these next exercises.

Exercise 9: Speak Healing Words (write your responses here or in your journal).

Identify one *healing* thing you said about yourself or someone else recently.

_____

_____

If you did not say anything healing about yourself today, why or why not?

_____

_____

Think of one healing thing that you can say about yourself and write it down here.

_____

_____

How did saying that healing thing make you feel?

_____

_____

Now identify one *hurtful* thing that you said about yourself or someone else today.

_____

_____

Why did you say that *hurtful* thing?

_____

_____

Now consider one thing you can do/say that could help you say something healing, either about yourself or the person you said something hurtful about.

_____

_____

Try to change your thoughts to healing thoughts and words into healing words. Hurtful words are more hurtful to us than the person we are speaking about. They are almost like a drug. We may feel good when we say them, but they become addictive over time and activate emotions that trigger a negative stress response. Not unlike when we eat junk food. It is pleasant while we are eating it, we become addicted to it, but it puts a lot of negative stress on our bodies.

Speaking healing words means that we have to change our thoughts from destructive thoughts to healing thoughts that activate the positive stress response and bring us closer to the net-positive stress zone.

It can also change our life conditions. The book As a Man Thinketh by James Allen, as you might imagine, is about the importance of thoughts and how they shape our lives. If you look at your life, the condition you are in can more than likely be related to the thoughts you feed yourself about yourself and others regularly. Change your thoughts, change your life condition. Start speaking healing words today!

This Cost Nothing Financially

Practicing the exercises in this chapter costs nothing yet could help us improve our food choices and health in a profound way. Let's move on to some more popular stress management techniques in the next chapter.

CHAPTER 20

MORE STRESS MANAGEMENT TECHNIQUES

The previous chapter was all about mental techniques that help put us in the net-positive stress zone. This chapter focuses on physical techniques that help put us in the net-positive stress zone. Remember to relax and take things step by step; everything does not need to be done at once.

Stress Management Technique #7: Exercise

Many of the centenarians that live in the Blue Zones mentioned earlier get their exercise "naturally." Not through gym memberships and stressful workouts. They may walk up and down stairs regularly, grow and harvest food, walk to and from work, etc. Consider incorporating more exercise into your life. It is powerful stress relief for our bodies, and it provides a host of other benefits. Here are some of these benefits:

- ☑ Reduces stress (brings us closer to that net-positive stress zone)
- ☑ Allows us to blow off steam (another way to reduce stress)
- ☑ Increases energy levels
- ☑ Puts us in a better mood
- ☑ Helps with memory and attention levels

- ☑ It's a powerful way to control blood sugar
- ☑ Circulates blood/oxygen throughout the body (this helps body organs and hormonal systems to function optimally)
- ☑ Prevents and relieves arthritis pain
- ☑ Builds muscle
- ☑ Burns calories and increases metabolism, which is helpful for weight management
- ☑ Helps us to sleep better

Ways to Incorporate Exercise into Your Life at No Cost

If you can get some form of aerobics (the exercise that gets you huffing and puffing), stretching, and weight-bearing activity into your week, that is the ultimate exercise goal. Start out small with one or two minutes a day and work your way up. The recommendation is 30 minutes a day. Here are some ways to get started:

Aerobic Exercise
- ☑ Take a power walk during your work break.
- ☑ Take the stairs at work or in your apartment complex/condo.
- ☑ Park further away from wherever you are going and walk.
- ☑ Walk around the house while you are on the phone.
- ☑ If you have a bike, start riding it more.
- ☑ Do yard work/mow the lawn.
- ☑ Power clean your place regularly.
- ☑ Dance to your favorite songs at home by yourself or with your family.
- ☑ Play outside with your kids.
- ☑ Find a 3-5-minute exercise video on the internet that you enjoy (Move your way up to 10, 15, or 20 minutes or more if you want to.).
- ☑ Create your own 3–5-minute exercise routine (Increase time intervals over time.).

Weight Bearing Activities
- ☑ Leg lifts and arm curls with weights while watching TV or on the phone.
- ☑ While cooking, stop periodically and lift a heavier pot you are not using up and down a few times.
- ☑ Do some gardening or landscaping at your home or around your apartment (many find it to be therapeutic).

Stretching
- ☑ If you work at a desk, stand up every 20-30 minutes and stretch or walk around for one minute.
- ☑ Do a two-minute stretch routine while deep breathing when you wake up and/or before you go to bed (find a YouTube video if you need a routine).

Anything that gets the body moving and the blood flowing counts as exercise. Even five extra minutes a day can make a difference.

Stress Management Technique #8: Sleep

Another way to move us closer to a net-positive stress zone is to get a good night's sleep. A good sleep is like a rejuvenating love letter to your body. And you deserve to receive that love letter *every night*.

If you are having difficulties sleeping through the night, consider investing some time into figuring out why you are having these difficulties. Then, find ways to improve your sleep. It is recommended that we get 7-9 hours of sleep for optimal health. If your schedule does not permit that, then that is all the more reason to make sure the sleep that you are able to get is amazing. The benefits of sleep are just as immense as those of exercise (and exercise helps us get better sleep).

Here are just a few benefits of good sleep:[80]
- ☑ Helps balance hunger hormones, making you less hungry throughout the day.

- ☑ Decreases risk of heart disease and obesity.
- ☑ Gives you more energy throughout the day.
- ☑ Helps fight infections like cold, flu, and COVID.
- ☑ Helps control blood sugar levels.
- ☑ Can improve learning and problem-solving skills.
- ☑ Promotes a better mood.
- ☑ Leads to more productivity.
- ☑ Decrease the risk of accidents.

Some things you can do to help you get a good night's sleep include:

- ☑ Avoid eating 3-4 hours before going to bed.
- ☑ Choose a bedtime and stick to it.
- ☑ Read a few book pages instead of using a screen before bed.
- ☑ Stretch and take 10-20 deep breaths before going to bed.
- ☑ If you can cool the room down, do it.
- ☑ Make the room as dark as possible.
- ☑ Cancel the negative thoughts and worries.
- ☑ Reduce noise or use white noise and headphones.
- ☑ If you have pain, see if diet or exercise can help. For example, eating omega-3s and doing exercise can provide arthritis pain relief. Some people even find pain relief from something as simple as drinking more water.
- ☑ Medication timing (ask your doctor if you can change your medication time to see if it helps you sleep better).
- ☑ If you think you have a sleep disorder, see a doctor.

From my experience, not canceling negative thoughts and worries is one of the main reasons many of us can't get a good night's sleep. This is why Chapter 19 is so important. Mental health impacts our physical health in so many ways. Some of you are rightfully worried about your job, your children, your family, your health, your finances, and the list goes on. You then bring that worry to the pillow. Go back to Chapter 19 if you have to. Some of the exercises can help.

The following stress management techniques can also help you get a good night's sleep and bring you closer to the net-positive stress zone.

Stress Management Technique #9: Deep Breathing
1. Take a slow, deep breath through your nose.
2. Count to five while breathing in—1, 2, 3, 4, 5.
3. Hold it for three seconds—1, 2, 3.
4. Breathe out slowly through your mouth.
5. Count to seven while breathing out—1, 2, 3, 4, 5, 6, 7.
6. Repeat several times.

If you've ever taken an exercise or stretching class or watched an exercise video, you may have heard the instructor say, "take a deep breath." One reason they say that is because taking those deep breaths on top of the exercise helps to circulate blood and, therefore, oxygen throughout the body better. The more we get blood and oxygen to the various places they need to be in the body, the better our organs and hormonal systems work.

While taking deep breaths when exercising and stretching is great, you can also take deep breaths wherever you are and no matter what you are doing. You can take deep breaths in the car with the kids in there (you can even do it with your kids), at work, during a meeting, in bed, while watching TV, or reading a book.

Imagine taking deep breaths and afterward giving yourself a statement of grace (see chapter 19). It can help reduce stress right at the moment and help with anxiety, which can result in better sleep and less stress. And closer to the net positive stress zone we go. Let's continue with more stress management.

Stress Management Technique #10: Prayer or Meditation

Prayer and meditation can be very calming forces in our lives because they create time for stopping, refocusing our thoughts, and shifting them in a direction that can promote a positive stress response. Several people from a variety of religions attribute healing and relief from anxiety to these simple practices. There is no right or wrong way to pray or meditate, but here is a loose definition of each:

Prayer involves communicating with God or other worshipped beings, usually in order to express gratitude, worship, ask for guidance or help, and achieve enlightenment.

Meditation involves focusing our minds on the present, often through breathing, and removing distracting thoughts. This is done to connect with our true nature, achieve inner peace, contentment, gratitude in life, and enlightenment.

Prayer and meditation pull together many stress management techniques mentioned. Taking a minute or two out of our day to pray or meditate can open the door to several other stress relievers. For example, as you meditate and pray, you can take deep breaths. They can also lead to gratefulness, giving ourselves grace, and speaking healing words, as discussed in Chapter 19.

In the end, we are positioning ourselves to improve our health through reduced inflammation, blood pressure and blood sugar control, and much more. But also, we are positioning ourselves to make choices (including our food choices) out of a more peaceful state of mind.

We may have a food system that throws its unhealthy and addictive food concoctions in our faces every chance it gets, and we might find what they are selling hard to resist every moment of every day. However, stopping to practice these stress management techniques can be just what we need to offset their influence in our lives. It can help us regain control in a world where things seem out of control and out of reach.

There are several other things you can do to manage stress that I won't go into as much depth about, but they can also be very helpful for our mental and physical health.

Other Stress Management Techniques:
- ☑ Reading
- ☑ Journaling
- ☑ Listening to music
- ☑ Laughter
- ☑ Learning to say "No"
- ☑ Going outside and enjoying the fresh air
- ☑ Volunteering
- ☑ Therapy (sometimes our insurance/jobs cover therapy sessions, inquire to see if that is the case for you)
- ☑ Download a stress management app
- ☑ Take a mental health day from work
- ☑ Do some gardening (see chapter 21)
- ☑ Listen to calming or inspirational music
- ☑ Do a puzzle
- ☑ Paint a picture or color in a coloring book
- ☑ Arts, crafts, and other activities with family
- ☑ Call a friend/family member

There are many other ways to manage stress. Figure out what works for you and move toward that net-positive stress zone until you achieve it. Remember to take things step by step and to avoid overwhelming yourself by doing too much at once. You will find a balance that is right for you, starting with deciding your commitment (See Chapter 11 for more on setting realistic goals and making a commitment.).

Now, let's find more stress relief from resources that are out there to help us achieve our health goals.

PART 4

THE SUPPORT
RESOURCES AVAILABLE FOR YOU

CHAPTER 21

FOOD ASSISTANCE AND OTHER RESOURCES

If you are eligible, there are some great resources available that can help defray some of your food costs. Some may require more effort than is desirable, but in many cases, they are worth the effort. Take advantage of these resources if you can.

Government Assistance

The Supplemental Nutrition Assistance Program (SNAP)

According to the United States Department of Agriculture website, "SNAP provides food benefits to low-income families to supplement their grocery budget so they can afford the nutritious food essential to health and well-being."[81]

If you are eligible and apply, you will receive a monthly stipend in the form of a Electronic Benefits Transfer (or EBT) card to use toward food at participating stores. Most grocery stores and other stores that sell food accept SNAP dollars, and several online vendors even accept SNAP now.

Even though it is a supplement and not designed to cover our entire food budget, for many, it is worth the effort it takes to apply. Even if it just covers your monthly fruit and vegetable budget.

Eligibility:
- ☑ Income-based

For Information on How to Apply:
- ☑ Visit https://www.fns.usda.gov/snap/state-directory or,
- ☑ Do an internet search for "How to apply for SNAP" or,
- ☑ Your local food bank will likely have information.

Women Infants and Children (WIC)

WIC is a food assistance program for women, infants, and children up to age five. According to their website: "Women, Infants, and Children (WIC) provides federal grants to states for supplemental foods, health care referrals, and nutrition education for low-income pregnant, breastfeeding, and non-breastfeeding postpartum women, and to infants and children up to age 5 who are found to be at nutritional risk."[82]

If you are eligible and apply, you will receive at no financial cost to you:
- ☑ Food staples like milk, whole grain bread, pasta, peanut butter, eggs, beans, cereals, yogurt, and more (For a complete list of WIC-eligible foods, visit the WIC website or do an internet search for WIC-eligible foods.)
- ☑ Nutrition counseling
- ☑ Health screenings
- ☑ Referrals to other health and social services

It is a great program that has proven itself to be effective at preventing nutrient deficiencies and health problems associated with those deficiencies.

Eligibility:
- ☑ Income-based
- ☑ Pregnant, breastfeeding, post-partum
- ☑ Infants and toddlers (up to 5 years old)
- ☑ Nutrition need is assessed

For Information on How to Apply:
- ☑ Visit https://www.fns.usda.gov/wic/program-contacts or,
- ☑ Do an internet search for "How to apply for WIC" or,
- ☑ Your local food bank more than likely will have information.

The Emergency Food Assistance Program (TEFAP)

TEFAP is another government program that provides monthly groceries to eligible individuals. According to its website, "The Emergency Food Assistance Program (TEFAP) is a federal program that helps supplement the diets of people with low income by providing them with emergency food assistance at no cost. USDA provides 100% American-grown USDA Foods and administrative funds to states to operate TEFAP."[83]

It is different from SNAP in that you do not receive a food stipend that you can use to purchase food. Instead, the foods you receive come from a food pantry or community-based meal setting (like a soup kitchen).

Eligibility:
- ☑ Income-based

For Information on How to Apply:
- ☑ Visit https://www.fns.usda.gov/tefap/program-contacts or,
- ☑ Do an internet search for "How to apply for TEFAP" or,
- ☑ Your local food bank more than likely will have information.

The Commodity Supplemental Food Program (CSFP)

According to the United States Department of Agriculture, "The Commodity Supplemental Food Program (CSFP) works to improve the health of low-income persons at least 60 years of age by supplementing their diets with nutritious USDA Foods. USDA distributes both food and administrative funds to participating states and Indian Tribal Organizations to operate CSFP."[84]

Participants receive food monthly that they can pick up from a food bank site or other distribution location. The food packages include oats, beans, rice, canned salmon, canned fruits, canned vegetables, and more.

Eligibility:
- ☑ Income-based
- ☑ Age-based (60 years or older)
- ☑ There may be other requirements depending on the state/territory

For Information on How to Apply:
- ☑ Visit https://www.fns.usda.gov/csfp/program-contacts or,
- ☑ Do an internet search for "How to apply for CSFP" or,
- ☑ Your local food bank (see Chapter 2) more than likely will have information.

The Senior Farmers Market Nutrition Program (SFMNP)

Per their website, "The Seniors Farmers Market Nutrition Program is designed to provide low-income seniors with access to locally grown fruits, vegetables, honey and herbs."[85]

This program provides anywhere from $20 to $40 a month in farmers' market dollars that you can use to purchase fresh produce at farmers' markets.

Eligibility:
- ☑ Income-based
- ☑ Age-based (60 years or older)

For Information on How to Apply:
- ☑ Visit https://www.fns.usda.gov/sfmnp/program-contacts or,
- ☑ Do an internet search for "How to apply for SFMNP" or,
- ☑ Your local food bank more than likely will have information.

Temporary Assistance to Needy Families Program (TANF)

TANF is a program that provides cash assistance to families and services that will help put them on a path to success. Services like employment programs, childcare subsidies, and mental health support. Per their website, "States use TANF to fund monthly cash assistance payments to low-income families with children, as well as a wide range of services."[86] You or somebody you know may be eligible for these payments and services.

Eligibility:
- ☑ Income-based
- ☑ Must have children
- ☑ Varies by state

For Information on How to Apply:
- ☑ Visit https://www.acf.hhs.gov/ofa/map/about/help-families or,
- ☑ Do an internet search for "How to apply for TANF" or,
- ☑ Your local food bank will likely have information.

SUN Bucks

There are seasonal programs to look out for like the SUN Bucks program. Per the USDA website "SUN Bucks is a new grocery benefit available across most of the U.S. Families with eligible school-aged children can get $120 per child to buy groceries during the summer."[87]

Eligibility:
- ☑ Income-based
- ☑ Age-based (school-aged children)
- ☑ Children must be enrolled in a school with a National School Lunch Program
- ☑ Automatically enrolled if you receive SNAP or TANF
- ☑ Other

For Information on How to Apply:
- ☑ Visit https://www.fns.usda.gov/summer/sunbucks to find the contact information for your state. Please note that some states do not participate in the program.

Food Banks

On top of hosting food distributions throughout the regions in which they are located, food banks provide food for food pantries at a largely discounted (or no) cost. Also, many of the government programs I mentioned, like TEFAP and CSFP, are run through food banks. The government provides the funding, and they run the show. For the food for programs that are not government funded, food banks rely on donations.

Over the past few years, there has been a shift to providing more nutritious and culturally relevant foods, so it's not just beans and rice anymore. So, how can you access the services that food banks have to offer?

Food Pantries

Food banks provide nonprofit organizations, including houses of worship, foods that they in turn distribute to the community. The best way to find a food pantry near you is to visit the website or call the food bank near you, which you can find at the Feeding America website, www.feedingamerica.org (See Chapter 2 for more information.). They provide a great variety of healthy foods *for anyone* that can help offset food costs significantly.

Weekly/Monthly Food Giveaways

On top of providing food to local non-profits, food banks often distribute food directly to the community through food giveaways. These are often places you can go to pick up food. Again, you can contact your local food bank to learn more about when and where these giveaways happen near you.

School/Summer Meals Programs

Food banks often provide meals to schools during the summer and at other times. Call the food bank in your area to find out if this service is available for you and your children.

Food Bank Nutrition Resources

More and more food banks have taken it upon themselves to provide nutrition information to the people they serve. Here are some nutrition services that a food bank near you may provide:
- ☑ Affordable recipes
- ☑ Nutrition classes
- ☑ Cooking classes
- ☑ Nutrition counseling with a dietitian

Gardening Resources

Some food banks also have a community teaching garden. Growing food is a therapeutic, healthy, and fun way to save money on food. Here are some resources that are typically available at some food banks to help get you started.
- ☑ Gardening classes
- ☑ Seed and seedling giveaways
- ☑ Garden starter kits include soil, pots, seeds, and other resources to start your garden.

Medically Tailored Meals/Food Services

There is a movement towards medically tailored meals. These meals are prepared for individuals with specific health conditions like heart disease, diabetes, and kidney disease to help manage them.

Eligible individuals can sign up for the meals, which are then delivered to their homes.

Several of these services are provided by non-profit organizations, which means that if you are eligible, you don't have to pay a dime for the meals. The nonprofit organization Food and Friends, located in Washington DC, for example, provides these meals to individuals who have been referred by their doctor, and there is no income requirement. They also provide nutrition counseling and a host of other services to ensure that individuals are getting the nutrition they need.

Eligibility:
- ☑ Differs by program

To Find a Medically Tailored Meals Program Near You:
- ☑ Visit the Food Is Medicine Coalition website at https://fimcoalition.org/find-agency/. Please note that several regions do not have the program, as it is a relatively new concept.

Your Doctor's Office or the Hospital

Some doctors, nurses, and other team members have information about resources and programs near you that can support you in your journey. Ask about it next time you go to the doctor. I mentioned the food delivery organization that delivers food specific to your health condition (medically tailored meals/food) as one resource.

There are also food prescription programs where you get a prescription for produce from your doctor that you can redeem at participating grocery stores (see below). There are several innovative ways healthy food is making its way into the health care system. Inquire about them.

Food Prescription Programs

As mentioned some doctors provide prescriptions for food at local participating supermarkets? For example, the Produce RX program run by the nonprofit organization DC Greens "allows medical professionals to prescribe fresh fruits and vegetables to DC Medicaid-enrolled patients who are experiencing a diet-related chronic illness"[88] These programs are few and far between, but they do exist, and they are very helpful for the individuals who use them. Ask your doctor if there are any programs in the area available to you.

Food Pharmacies

Some hospitals have what are called food pharmacies. These are spaces you can go in the hospital to receive food. Depending on the food pharmacy, most, if not all, of the food is healthy, and they even provide fresh produce sometimes. Ask your doctor if one is at your local hospital or doctor's office.

Create the Demand for Resources

The more people ask about these resources, the more of a demand you can create. There are millions of others who are dealing with similar issues, and you will not be alone in your request. If everyone who was in need asked for them, most doctors' offices would recognize the need for it and begin to provide this type of information if they did not provide it already.

Gardening Tips and Resources

Gardening is a fantastic way to save money. Fresh herbs can be very expensive but growing them yourself allows you to have a seasonal supply for as little as $3.00-$10.00, depending on how fancy you want to be with your containers. You can also grow things like tomatoes, onions, peppers, kale, collard greens, and the list goes on. I had no idea how much you could grow until I started a container garden on our deck. I learned to do this from my students who were also growing food in their front and back yards and inside their apartments.

We didn't have to buy certain food items for the entire season because they just kept growing. Even if we ate the entire plant, they would return within weeks. Some of the food (mostly peppers and tomatoes) grew so much that we had to give some away. And we are not growing on that big of a space.

To do basic gardening, you only need a pot/reusable food container, soil, seeds, and water. Don't have the money for soil and seeds? There are local non-profits that provide all kinds of gardening resources, including soil, seeds, and gardening classes at no cost.

To Find Gardening Resources Near You:
1. Contact your local food bank; they may have resources.
2. Do an internet search for "gardening non-profits near me."
3. Call your local botanical garden or arboretum.
4. Do an internet search for "community gardens near me."

Community gardens are great ways to get involved in a social group or get information about growing your own food. Gardening is also a great family activity. If you want to start gardening today, here are a few easy instructions:

Growing Tips

If you are new to growing, I recommend starting with easy-to-grow herbs like:
- ☑ Mint (for refreshing mint water and watermelon mint salad)
- ☑ Rosemary and thyme (for delicious roasted potatoes)
- ☑ Basil (for spaghetti sauce or homemade pesto)

To Grow a Seedling Plant (recommended if you are just starting out):
1. Find seedlings (seedlings are young plants) or herb plants at your local grocery store, nursery, or local nonprofit organization.
2. Find a sunny place where you can put the plant.

3. Water the seedling.
    a. Most plants do well when you just keep the soil damp (not soaking wet). Every day, I touch the soil and make sure it is damp, if it is not damp, I add enough water to make it damp.
    b. Seedlings are very forgiving, so if you think you are overwatering, they will tell you by how they look. They will also tell you if you are underwatering. It is important to pay attention to how they react with different water amounts.
    c. You can also find tips for watering your specific seedling/herb online.
4. Watch it grow.
5. Harvest and eat regularly when it is ready.
    a. The more you harvest and eat, the healthier the plant will be and the more food you will be able to grow.

To Grow from Seed

Growing from the seed of the plant is more difficult than growing from a seedling plant, and I would not recommend it for beginners unless you take a gardening class or watch educational videos. It also usually requires starting at a specific time of year, depending on what part of the country you live in. I live in Maryland, and I start my seeds in February to prepare them for the spring and summer. Nonetheless, if you want to be adventurous (or perhaps you can challenge your children to be), here is a way to get started:
1. Find a container
    a. Any container will do. It can be a milk carton, an unused planter you have lying around the house, a glass pickle jar, etc.
        i. For multiple seeds, there are tiny seed starter pots you can purchase. They cost $5 for twenty,

thirty, or even fifty pots. Once the seeds germinate and eventually grow into a seedling, you can transplant that seedling to a larger container.
   b. If you are growing herbs, you only need a small container. You will want a large container if you are growing tomatoes, peppers, or collard greens. The bigger the container, the bigger they will get.
2. Find a place where you can get soil and seeds.
   a. Again, find out if there are any nonprofits or community gardens near you for free resources.
3. Put the soil in the container.
4. The seed packets will have instructions you can follow.

Enjoy the fruits of your labor.

* * *

Several resources are available for individuals and families who may need extra help. Take advantage of these resources as they can help to alleviate some stress. Also, as you know from chapters 19 and 20, the more you are able to manage stress, the more likely you are to make better choices for your health and life.

CHAPTER 22

PUTTING IT ALL TOGETHER

I remember teaching a nutrition class at a community center, and a man said, "You are trying to tell us what we can and can't eat." While that was not my intention, I recognized that it could come off that way. This is why I have intentionally reminded you of that throughout this entire book. I told him that I was just providing information and that anybody listening (or reading, in this case) could take it or leave it.

Here are some things I hope you took away from this book:
- ☑ Food is intertwined with every aspect of our lives. So much so that it is difficult to achieve sustainable, healthy food lifestyle changes without making changes to our mental, emotional, and spiritual health (chapters 19-20).
- ☑ Healthy eating is possible even on a budget because whole plant-based foods often cost as much as or less than unhealthy foods (chapters 2-10).
- ☑ Setting goals, making commitments, and taking things step by step is the key to success for many (chapter 11).
- ☑ Understanding our nutrition needs is empowering and helpful for achieving our health goals (chapters 12-18).

- ☑ Stress management is just as important to our health as diet (chapters 19-20).
- ☑ Stress impacts the way we digest food and influences our food choices (chapters 19-20).
- ☑ The net-positive stress zone is possible to achieve (chapters 19-20).
- ☑ Problem-solving and asking for help are powerful ways to relieve stress (chapter 19).
- ☑ Your thoughts and how you talk about yourself can also relieve stress (chapter 19).
- ☑ There are several physical things you can do to relieve stress at no financial cost to you (chapter 20).
- ☑ There are resources available to help defray the cost of food (chapter 21).
- ☑ Gardening is a fun, cost-effective way to get exercise, have family time, and get the freshest and tastiest whole foods around town (chapter 21).

By practicing these activities and using the knowledge you received from this book regularly, you will also see other areas of your life improve. It all works together for good.

I am a dietitian; I have lived and breathed nutrition for the past twenty years…and I am still working on improving my diet. However, I get better with it year after year, and the changes I made have allowed me to manage my health condition so that I don't have to take medications and suffer from the symptoms. This allows me to live life to the fullest. It would be nice to be perfect, but then we wouldn't be human. So, stay encouraged on your journey and remember to keep moving forward no matter what. Little by little or lot by lot, you will achieve your goals.

ENDNOTES

Introduction
1. Please note that "diet" drinks won't make much of a positive difference. See Chapter 14 for more on this.
2. Cook HE, Garris LA, Gulum AH, et.al. Impact of SMART Goals on Diabetes Management in a Pharmacist-Led Telehealth Clinic. Journal of Pharmacy Practice. 2024;37(1):54-59. doi:10.1177/08971900221125021
3. Food Safety and Inspection Service. Safe Minimum Internal Temperature Chart. https://www.fsis.usda.gov/food-safety/safe-food-handling-and-preparation/food-safety-basics/safe-temperature-chart

Chapter 1: Easy Food Preparation Methods
4. Grdeń P, Jakubczyk A. Health Benefits of Legume Seeds. J Sci Food Agric, 2023;103(11):5213-5220. doi:10.1002/jsfa.12585
5. Li P, Hu Y, Zhan L, He J, et.al. A Natural Glucan from Black Bean Inhibits Cancer Cell Proliferation via PI3K-Akt and MAPK Pathway. Molecules. 2023 Feb 19;28(4):1971. doi: 10.3390/molecules28041971.

Chapter 2: Food Savings Pro Tips
6. Information from Seattle Public Utilities. https://www.seattle.gov/util/cs/groups/public/@spu/@conservation/documents/webcontent/1_037049.pdf, Accessed, 17 July 2024. They also have a fantastic website with lots of good information on waste prevention https://www.seattle.gov/utilities/protecting-our-environment/sustainability-tips/waste-prevention
7. Ibid.
8. Image from Illinois Extension. Save Money with Unit Pricing. https://eat-move-save.extension.illinois.edu/tour/grocery-store-tour/save-money-unit-pricing Accessed, 16 August 2024
9. Agency for Toxic Substances and Disease Registry. What are the health effects of PFAS? https://www.atsdr.cdc.gov/pfas/health_effects/index.html Accessed, 17 July 2024

10. U.S. Food and Drug Administration. Bottled Water Everywhere: Keeping it Safe https://www.fda.gov/consumers/consumer-updates/bottled-water-everywhere-keeping-it-safe Accessed, 22 August 2024
11. Anh NH, Kim SJ, Long NP, et al. Ginger on Human Health: A Comprehensive Systematic Review of 109 Randomized Controlled Trials. Nutrients. 2020; 12(1):157. doi: 10.3390/nu12010157.
12. Katz DL, Doughty K, Ali A. Cocoa and Chocolate in Human Health and Disease. Antioxid Redox Signal. 2011;15(10):2779-811. doi: 10.1089/ars.2010.3697.
13. Ibid.

Chapter 5: Snacks

14. Wallace TC, Bailey RL, Blumberg, et al. Fruits, Vegetables, and Health: A Comprehensive Narrative, Umbrella Review of the Science and Recommendations for Enhanced Public Policy to Improve Intake. Critical Reviews in Food Science and Nutrition. 2019;60(13):2174-2211. doi: 10.1080/10408398.2019.1632258
15. Yang H, Tian T, Wu D, et.al. Prevention and treatment effects of edible berries for three deadly diseases: Cardiovascular disease, cancer and diabetes. Crit Rev Food Sci Nutr. 2019;59(12):1903-1912. doi: 10.1080/10408398.2018.1432562
16. Rajaram S, Jones J, Lee GJ. Plant-Based Dietary Patterns, Plant Foods, and Age-Related Cognitive Decline. Adv Nutr. 2019;10(Suppl_4):S422-S436. doi:10.1093/advances/nmz081
17. Rahmani AH, Aly SM, Ali H, et al. Therapeutic Effects of Date Fruits (Phoenix dactylifera) in the Prevention of Diseases via Modulation of Anti-inflammatory, Antioxidant and Anti-tumour activity. Int J Clin Exp Med. 2014;7(3):483-491.
18. Harvard T.H. Chan School of Public Health. Avocados. https://www.hsph.harvard.edu/nutritionsource/avocados/ Accessed, 29 July 2024
19. I was in Costa Rica years ago, so things might have changed significantly, especially with the globalization of the standard American diet.

Chapter 8: Dinner

20. Smith HA, Betts JA. Nutrient Timing and Metabolic Regulation, The Journal of Physiology. 2022;600(6):1299-1312. doi: 10.1113/JP280756
21. Hamada Y, Hayashi N. Chewing increases postprandial diet-induced thermogenesis [published correction appears in Sci Rep. 2021 Dec 23;11(1):24483. doi: 10.1038/s41598-021-04257-w]. Sci Rep. 2021;11(1):23714. Published 2021 Dec 9. doi:10.1038/s41598-021-03109-x
22. Appel LJ, Foti K. Sources of Dietary Sodium: Implications for Patients, Physicians, and Policy. Circulation. 2017 May 9;135(19):1784-1787. doi: 10.1161/CIRCULATIONAHA.117.027933
23. Farvid MS, Sidahmed E, Spence ND, et al. Consumption of red meat and processed meat and cancer incidence: a systematic review and meta-analysis of prospective studies. Eur J Epidemiol. 2021;36(9):937-951. doi:10.1007/s10654-021-00741-9

Chapter 12: Calories

24. Flanagan EW, Most J, Mey JT, Redman LM. Calorie Restriction and Aging in Humans. Annu Rev Nutr. 2020;40:105-133. doi:10.1146/annurev-nutr-122319-034601
25. Food and Nutrition Board, Institute of Medicine, National Academies. Dietary Reference Intakes (DRIs): Acceptable Macronutrient Distribution Ranges. https://www.ncbi.nlm.nih.gov/books/NBK56068/table/summarytables.t5/?report=objectonly

26. Arif Icer M, Acar Tek N. Effects of Red Pepper, Ginger, and Turmeric on Energy Metabolism: Review of Current Knowledge. Altern Ther Health Med. 2023;29(3):81-87.https://pubmed.ncbi.nlm.nih.gov/33789250/
27. Ibid.
28. Ibid.
29. Faria NC, Soares APDC, Graciano GF et al. Acute green tea infusion ingestion effect on energy metabolism, satiety sensation and food intake: A randomized crossover trial. Clin Nutr ESPEN. 2022;48:63-67. doi:10.1016/j.clnesp.2022.01.034
30. Mu WJ, Zhu JY, Chen M, Guo L. Exercise-Mediated Browning of White Adipose Tissue: Its Significance, Mechanism and Effectiveness. Int J Mol Sci. 2021;22(21):11512. Published 2021 Oct 26. doi:10.3390/ijms222111512
31. Depner CM, Stothard ER, Wright KP Jr. Metabolic consequences of sleep and circadian disorders. Curr Diab Rep. 2014;14(7):507. doi:10.1007/s11892-014-0507-z

Chapter 13: Decoding the Mysteries of the Nutrition Facts Label and Ingredients List

32. U.S. Food and Drug Administration Center for Food Safety and Applied Nutrition. A Food Labelling Guide (page 17). https://www.fda.gov/files/food/published/Food-Labeling-Guide-%28PDF%29.pdf Accessed, 16 August 2024
33. Image from U.S. Food and Drug Administration Center for Food Safety and Applied Nutrition. A Food Labelling Guide (page 23). https://www.fda.gov/files/food/published/Food-Labeling-Guide-%28PDF%29.pdf Accessed, 16 August 2024
34. Image from The U.S. Food and Drug Administration. Changes to the Nutrition Facts Label Panel. https://www.fda.gov/food/food-labeling-nutrition/changes-nutrition-facts-label Accessed, 16 August 2024
35. Image from The U.S. Food and Drug Administration. How to Understand and Use the Nutrition Facts Label https://www.fda.gov/food/nutrition-facts-label/how-understand-and-use-nutrition-facts-label Accessed, 16 August 2024
36. Image from The U.S. Food and Drug Administration. Interactive Nutrition Label. https://www.accessdata.fda.gov/scripts/InteractiveNutritionFactsLabel/#intro Accessed, 16 August 2024
37. Serving Size Question Answers
    1. 4 grams of total sugars.
    2. 16 grams of total sugars. The entire package contains four servings, so multiply four grams of sugar by four servings to get 16 grams.
    3. 6 grams of saturated fat. Don't forget that the entire package contains 4 servings so you must multiply 1.5 grams of saturated fat times 4 servings to get six grams.
    4. 12 milligrams of iron are in two servings (6 grams per serving x 2 servings = 12 grams).
    5. 3 cups are in two servings of this food item (1.5 cups x 2 servings).
38. Iizuka K. Is the Use of Artificial Sweeteners Beneficial for Patients with Diabetes Mellitus? The Advantages and Disadvantages of Artificial Sweeteners. Nutrients. 2022;14(21):4446. Published 2022 Oct 22. doi:10.3390/nu14214446
39. Ibid.
40. Ibid.
41. Image from the U.S. Food and Drug Administration. Interactive Nutrition Label – Sugar Alcohols. https://www.accessdata.fda.gov/scripts/InteractiveNutritionFactsLabel/assets/InteractiveNFL_SugarAlcohols_October2021.pdf Accessed, 28 August 2024

42. Witkowski M, Nemet I, Li XS, et al. Xylitol is prothrombotic and associated with cardiovascular risk European Heart Journal. 2024;45(27):2439–2452. doi:10.1093/eurheartj/ehae244

Chapter 14: Carbohydrates
43. % Daily Value Quiz Answers
    1. 19% of recommended sodium for the day.
    2. 57% of recommended sodium for the day (19% x 3 servings = 57%).
    3. 50% of recommended fiber for the day (25% x 2 servings = 50%).
    4. 6% of recommended potassium for the day.
44. National Institutes of Health Office of Dietary Supplements. Nutrient Recommendations and Databases. https://ods.od.nih.gov/HealthInformation/nutrientrecommendations.aspx Accessed, 16 June 2024
45. There is debate even around using the terms "healthy" and "unhealthy."
46. Ramsing R, Santo R, Kim BF, et al. Dairy and Plant-Based Milks: Implications for Nutrition and Planetary Health. Curr Environ Health Rep. 2023;10(3):291-302. doi:10.1007/s40572-023-00400-z
47. Ibid.
48. Skaaby T, Kilpeläinen TO, Mahendran Y, et al. Association of milk intake with hay fever, asthma, and lung function: a Mendelian randomization analysis. Eur J Epidemiol. 2022;37(7):713-722. doi:10.1007/s10654-021-00826-5

Chapter 15: Fats
49. Table from the National Institutes of Health. Body Mass Index Table 1. https://www.nhlbi.nih.gov/health/educational/lose_wt/BMI/bmi_tbl.htm Accessed, 16 August 2024
50. Antoni R. Dietary saturated fat and cholesterol: cracking the myths around eggs and cardiovascular disease. J Nutr Sci. 2023;12:e97. Published 2023 Sep 11. doi:10.1017/jns.2023.82
51. Ibid.
52. Ibid.
53. Mei J, Qian M, Hou Y, et al. Association of saturated fatty acids with cancer risk: a systematic review and meta-analysis. Lipids in Health and Disease. 2024;23:32. doi:10.1186/s12944-024-02025-z
54. Mostafa H, Gutierrez-Tordera L, Mateu-Fabregat J, et al. Dietary fat, telomere length and cognitive function: unravelling the complex relations. Curr Opin Lipidol. 2024; 35(1):33-40. doi:10.1097/MOL.0000000000000900
55. Ibid.
56. American Heart Association. Saturated Fat. https://www.heart.org/en/healthy-living/healthy-eating/eat-smart/fats/saturated-fats Accessed, 7 September 2024
57. Bafail D, Bafail A, Alshehri N, et.al. Impact of Coconut Oil and Its Bioactive Metabolites in Alzheimer's Disease and Dementia: A Systematic Review and Meta-Analysis. Diseases. 2024 Nov 1;12(11):272. doi: 10.3390/diseases12110272
58. De Oliveira e Silva ER, Seidman CE, et al. Effects of shrimp consumption on plasma lipoproteins. Am J Clin Nutr. 1996;64(5):712-717. doi:10.1093/ajcn/64.5.712
59. Antoni R. Dietary saturated fat and cholesterol: cracking the myths around eggs and cardiovascular disease. J Nutr Sci. 2023;12:e97. Published 2023 Sep 11. doi:10.1017/jns.2023.82

60. Farag MA, Gad MZ. Omega-9 fatty acids: potential roles in inflammation and cancer management. J Genet Eng Biotechnol. 2022;20(1):48. Published 2022 Mar 16. doi:10.1186/s43141-022-00329-0.
61. National Institutes of Health Office of Dietary Supplements. Omega 3 Fatty Acids Fact Sheet for Consumers. https://ods.od.nih.gov/factsheets/Omega3FattyAcids-Consumer/ Accessed, 13 June 2024
62. Ibid.
63. Dietary Reference Intakes (DRIs): Recommended Dietary Allowances and Adequate Intakes, Total Water and Macronutrients, https://www.ncbi.nlm.nih.gov/books/NBK56068/table/summarytables.t4/?report=objectonly Accessed, 16 March 2024
64. Kim HK, Kang EY, Go GW. Recent insights into dietary ω-6 fatty acid health implications using a systematic review. Food Sci Biotechnol. 2022;31(11):1365-1376. Published 2022 Aug 20. doi:10.1007/s10068-022-01152-6

Chapter 17: Vitamins, Minerals, and Phytonutrients
65. Waheed Janabi AH, Kamboh AA, Saeed M, et al. Flavonoid-rich foods (FRF): A promising nutraceutical approach against lifespan-shortening diseases. Iran J Basic Med Sci. 2020;23(2):140-153. doi:10.22038/IJBMS.2019.35125.8353
66. Terao J. Revisiting carotenoids as dietary antioxidants for human health and disease prevention Food Funct. 2023;14(17):7799-7824. doi:10.1039/D3FO02330C
67. Isemura M. Catechin in Human Health and Disease. Molecules. 2019;24(3):528. doi:10.3390/molecules24030528
68. Harvard Health Publishing Harvard Medical School. Time for more vitamin D. https://www.health.harvard.edu/staying-healthy/time-for-more-vitamin-d Accessed, 16 September 2024
69. Ibid.
70. Information from The U.S. Food and Drug Administration. Interactive Nutrition Facts Label – Vitamins and Minerals Chart. https://www.accessdata.fda.gov/scripts/InteractiveNutritionFactsLabel/assets/InteractiveNFL_Vitamins&MineralsChart_October2021.pdf Accessed, 16 August 2024
71. Ibid.

Chapter 18: Other Nutrition Questions Answered
72. U.S. Food and Drug Administration. How GMOs Are Regulated in the United States. https://www.fda.gov/food/agricultural-biotechnology/how-gmos-are-regulated-united-states#:~:text=The%20National%20Bioengineered%20Food%20Disclosure,breeding%20or%20found%20in%20nature Accessed, 23 July 2024
73. U.S. Food and Drug Administration. GMO Crops, Animal Food, and Beyond. https://www.fda.gov/food/agricultural-biotechnology/gmo-crops-animal-food-and-beyond Accessed, 23 July 2024
74. U.S. Department of Agriculture. List of Bioengineered Foods https://www.ams.usda.gov/rules-regulations/be/bioengineered-foods-list Accessed, 23 July 2024
75. U.S. Food and Drug Administration. Sodium in Your Diet Use the Nutrition Facts Label and Reduce Your Intake https://www.fda.gov/food/nutrition-education-resources-materials/sodium-your-diet#:~:text=Despite%20what%20many%20people%20think,food%20when%20cooking%20or%20eating Accessed, 23 August 2024

Chapter 19: Relax and Give Yourself a Break

76. Cherpak CE. Mindful Eating: A Review Of How The Stress-Digestion-Mindfulness Triad May Modulate And Improve Gastrointestinal And Digestive Function. Integr Med (Encinitas). 2019;18(4):48-53.
77. Girotti M, Adler SM, Bulin SE, et. al. Prefrontal cortex executive processes affected by stress in health and disease. Prog Neuropsychopharmacol Biol Psychiatry. 2018 Jul 13;85:161-179. doi: 10.1016/j.pnpbp.2017.07.004
78. NIH News in Health. Practicing Gratitude, Ways to Improve Positivity. https://newsinhealth.nih.gov/2019/03/practicing-gratitude Accessed, 20 September 2024
79. Harvard Health Publishing Harvard Medical School. Understanding The Stress Response, Chronic activation of this survival mechanism impairs health. https://www.health.harvard.edu/staying-healthy/understanding-the-stress-response Accessed, 23 September 2024

Chapter 20: More Stress Management Techniques

80. National Heart, Lung, and Blood Institute. Sleep Deprivation and Deficiency, How Sleep Affects Your Health. https://www.nhlbi.nih.gov/health/sleep-deprivation/health-effects Accessed, 27 September 2024

Chapter 21: Food Assistance and Other Resources

81. U.S. Department of Agriculture Food and Nutrition Service. Supplemental Nutrition Assistance Program. https://www.fns.usda.gov/snap/supplemental-nutrition-assistance-program Accessed, 11 June 2024
82. U.S. Department of Agriculture Food and Nutrition Service. Special Supplemental Nutrition Program for Women, Infants, and Children (WIC). https://www.fns.usda.gov/wic Accessed, 12 June 2024
83. U.S. Department of Agriculture Food and Nutrition Service. The Emergency Food Assistance Program. https://www.fns.usda.gov/tefap/emergency-food-assistance-program Accessed, 14 June 2024
84. U.S. Department of Agriculture Food and Nutrition Service. Commodity Supplemental Food Program. https://www.fns.usda.gov/csfp/commodity-supplemental-food-program Accessed, 16 June 2024
85. U.S. Department of Agriculture Food and Nutrition Service. Seniors Farmers Market Nutrition Program. https://www.fns.usda.gov/sfmnp/senior-farmers-market-nutrition-program Accessed, 17 June 2024
86. U.S. Department of Health & Human Services. Temporary Assistance for Needy Families (TANF). https://www.acf.hhs.gov/ofa/programs/temporary-assistance-needy-families-tanf Accessed, 17 June 2024
87. U.S. Department of Agriculture Food and Nutrition Service. SUN Bucks (Summer EBT) https://www.fns.usda.gov/summer/sunbucks Accessed, 11 July 2024
88. DC Greens Produce Rx Program https://dcgreens.org/produce-rx/?gad_source=1&gclid=CjwKCAiArva5BhBiEiwA-oTnXVTRdOGD7V6ScO5uXl5njaRqBZ0OJ4uDluadVYsIGAUoFqYhrr1DUhoCXSwQAvD_BwE Accessed, 11 October 2024

INDEX

A
Added sugars, 172, 174
Agave, 177
Aging, 78
    And Berries, 79
    And Calories, 158
    And Coconut Oil, 217
    And Saturated Fats, 211
    Foods that Reduce Age-
        Related Disease Risk, 79
Air fryers, 21
Alcohol
    Calories From, 155
Antioxidants, 239
Applesauce
    Homemade, 80
Artificial sweeteners, 175
Avocado
    Homemade Guacamole, 88
    Snack, 87
    Ways to Enjoy, 88

B
Baking, 20, 21
Bananas, 77
Basal Metabolic Rate, 157
Beans
    With Rice and Steamed
        Veggies, 128
Beans and Rice
    Homemade and Easy, 103
Berries, 78
Best By Dates, 53
Black Bean
    Patties/Burgers, 120
    With Homemade French
        Fries, 120
Body Mass Index (BMI), 208
Breakfast, 99

C
Calcium, 247
Calories
    And Aging, 158
    How Many For Me?, 156
    Overview, 155
    Sources, 155
    What Are They?, 155
Carbohydrates
    Calories From, 155

322 ■ AFFORDABLE HEALTHY FOOD

Carb Loading, 195
Conflicting Views, 201
Dry to Cook conversions, 191
Good vs. Bad, 195
How Many Do We Need?, 187
How To Find, 190
Net Carbs, 191
On Nutrition Facts Panel, 172
Simple vs. Complex, 184
Sources, 185
What Are They?, 183
Chewing Your Food, 261
Chia Seeds
    Health Benefits, 106
    Homemade Pudding, 106
Children
    100% Juices, 68
    Applesauce, 80
    As Helpers, 273
    Chili, 126
    Egg Muffins, 104
    Generic Brands, 48
    Government Support
        (Sunbucks), 305
    Government Support
        (TANF), 305
    Government Support (WIC),
        302
    Growing Herbs, 54
    Homemade Vegan Pizza, 132
    Oatmeal Bites, 101
    Smoothies, 83
    Snacking Vegetables, 86
    Tacos, 113
Chili
    Homemade, Vegetarian, 126
Cholesterol
    Eggs, 219
    Foods That Increase, 219

HDL Vs. LDL, 218
Healthy Vs. Unhealthy, 218
Overview, 218
Shrimp, 219
Cocoa and Cacao Powder, 71
Cocoa/Cacao
    Health Benefits, 71
    What is the Difference?), 71
Coconut Oil, 216
Collard Green
    Wrap, 116
Community Gardens, 310
Cooking Basics, 15
Cooking Methods
    Overview, 11
Corn
    Corn on the Cob, 95
    Health Benefits, 95
Cottage Cheese, 93
Cravings
    Trick for Sweet, 110

D

Dates, 85
Diet, 7, 149, 319
Dinner, 119
Drinks, 61

E

Eating Out on a Budget, 137
Eggs
    Homemade Egg Muffins, 104
    Scrambled with Avocado, 105

F

Fats
    Calories From, 155
    Coconut Oil, 216
    Common Sources, 226

Fish, 226
Good Vs. Bad, 211
Mono-Unsaturated ('Good' fats), 222
Omega-3s ('Good' fats), 223
Overview, 207
Saturated, 211
Trans, 220
Unsaturated, 222
Fiber
    Foods With, 198, 199
    Is a Carbohydrate, 185
Flaxseeds, 225
Food Assistance
    Medically Tailored Meals, 308
    Seasonal Programs, 305
    SNAP, 301
    The Commodity Supplemental Food Program (CSFP), 303
    The Emergency Food Assistance Program (TEFAP), 303
    The Senior Nutrition Farmers Market Program (SFMNP), 304
    The Temporary Assistance to Needy Families Program (TANF), 305
    WIC, 302
Food Banks
    And Food Giveaways, 306
    And Food Pantries, 306
    And Gardening Resources, 307
    And Nutrition Resources, 307
    And School/Summer Meals, 307
Food Distribution Centers, 37
Food Giveaways, 306

Food Log, 163
Food Pantries, 306
Food Pantry
    Near You, 37
Food Pharmacies, 309
Food Prep Challenge, 35
Food Prescription Programs, 308
Food Safety
    Cooking Temperatures, 16
    Washing Meat, 20
Food Synergy, 76
Frozen Foods/Meals, 140
Fruit
    Fruit Cups, 81
    Handheld, 79
    In Season, 77
Fruits and Vegetables
    As Snacks, 75
    Eat the Rainbow, 75

G

Gardening
    Tips and Resources, 309
Genetically Modified Organisms (GMOs), 251
Ginger, 70
Gluten
    Sources, 204
GMOs. *See* Genetically Modified Organisms
Government Assistance, 301
Grains
    Millet, 134
    Quinoa, 134
    Refined, 186
    Whole, 186
Guacamole
    Homemade, 88
    Ways to Eat, 88

H
HDL Cholesterol, 218
Herbs/Spice Combinations, 19
Homemade Hot Sauce, 132
Homemade Vegan Pizza, 132

I
Iceberg Lettuce, 95
Ingredients List, 165
Iron, 248

L
LDL Cholesterol, 218
Legumes, 32
Lentils
    Different types, 124
    Health Benefits, 124
    Soup, 124
Lentils and Rice, 125
Lettuce
    Wrap, 116
Lunch, 109

M
Magnesium, 248
Measuring Cups, 170
Meat Alternatives, 140
Medically Tailored Meals, 307
Metabolism, 161
    Definition, 161
    Foods that increase, 161
Microbiome, 78
Milk
    A2, 199
    Cows Vs. Plant-Based, 199
    Goat, 199
    Raw, 199
Millet
    For breakfast, 134
    Instead of rice, 134

Minerals
    Calcium, 247
    Chloride, 247
    Chromium, 247
    Copper, 248
    Iodine, 248
    Iron, 248
    Magnesium, 248
    Manganese, 249
    Molybdenum, 249
    Phosphorus, 249
    Potassium, 249
    Selenium, 249
    Sodium, 250
    Zinc, 250

N
Net Carbs, 191
Nutrient Quantities, 172
Nutrition Facts Label, 319
    Macronutrients (Fats, Carbs, and Protein), 172
    Micronutrients (Vitamins and Minerals), 172
    Overview, 165
    Percent Daily Value (%DV), 177
    Serving Size, 167
    Servings Per Container, 167

O
Oatmeal
    Homemade Oatmeal Bites, 101
    With Water, 100
Oils
    Overview, 227
    Smoke Point, 228
Omelet, Vegetarian, 131
Organic
    Is it Worth it?, 41

The Clean Fifteen, 41
The Dirty Dozen, 41

P

Peanut Butter
　Apples and Peanut Butter, 82
　Choosing Healthy, 82
　With Celery, 87
Peanuts, 91
Percent Daily Value (%DV), 177
Phytonutrients, 239
Pickling, 28
　Food Prep Challenge, 35
　How To, 28
Plantain
　Homemade chips, 96
Plant-Based Milk, 199
Popcorn, 90
Portion Control, 260
Potassium, 249
Potatoes
　Are Very Healthy, 95
　Baked Home Fries, 103
　Homemade Potato Chips, 94
　With Salsa, 94
Prebiotics, 78
Probiotics, 78
Protein
　Amino Acids, 231
　Calories From, 155
　Complete vs. Incomplete, 231
　How Much Do I Need?, 233
　How to Calculate, 233
　Overview, 231
　Plant-Based, 16
　Protein Powders, 236

R

Refined Grains, 186
Roasting/Baking, 19

S

Salad
　Combination Recommendations, 112
　Easy Homemade Dressing, 112
　Homemade, 110
Salt vs. Sodium, 256
Sautéing, 22
Savings, 37
Seasoning, 18
Selenium, 249
Serving Size
　As a Way to Save Money, 53
　Nutrition Facts Label, 167
Servings Per Container, 170
Slow Cooking, 27
Smoothies, 83
　For Breakfast, 108
Snacking Vegetables, 86
Snacks, 75
Sodium
　Function and Sources, 250
　How Much Per Day?, 254
　Salt, 254
　Salt Alternatives, 254
Spaghetti
　Homemade, Vegetarian, 127
Split Pea Soup, 123
Staple Foods, 57
Starches
　Are Carbohydrates, 185
　Foods With, 199
Steaming, 25
Stevia, 177
Storage Guide, 42, 43
Stress
　Activity, 270
　And Digestion, 268
　And Exercise, 291

And Food Choices, 269
And Gratitude, 284
And Guilt, 283
And Sleep, 293
Hormones, 267
Management, 268
Management Exercises, 285
Management Techniques, 273
Negative and Positive, 268
Types, 268
Stuffed Bell Peppers, 129
Sugar
    Foods With, 198
    Is a Carbohydrate, 185
    Strategy to Reduce, 72
Sugar Alcohols, 176
Sunflower Seeds, 91
Supplemental Nutrition Assistance Program (SNAP), 301
Supplements, 243
Sweet Potato
    Baked, 102

T

Tacos
    Homemade, 113
The Clean Fifteen, 41
The Commodity Supplemental Food Program (CSFP), 303
The Dirty Dozen, 41
The Emergency Food Assistance Program, 303
The Senior Nutrition Farmers Market Program (SFMNP), 304
The Temporary Assistance to Needy Families Program (TANF), 305

Trail Mix
    Homemade, 91
Trans Fats, 220
Tuna Fish
    Salad, 115
    With Veggies, 115

U

Unit Prices, 45

V

Vegetables
    In Season, 86
Vinaigrette
    Homemade Salad Dressing, 112
Vitamin B12
    And Vegan Diets, 123
Vitamin D
    Function and Sources, 246
    Overview, 241
Vitamins
    Biotin, 244
    Choline, 245
    Folate/Folic Acid (B9), 245
    Niacin (B3), 245
    Pantothenic Acid (B5), 245
    Riboflavin (B2), 245
    Thiamin (B1), 246
    Vitamin A, 246
    Vitamin B6, 246
    Vitamin B12, 246
    Vitamin C, 246
    Vitamin D, 246
    Vitamin E, 247
    Vitamin K, 247
Vitamins and Minerals
    Activity, 244
    Overview, 239

W
Water
 Bottled, 64
 Filters, 63
 Overview, 62
Water Filters, 63
Watermelon, 85
Weight Management, 257
Whole Grains, 186
Women, Infants and Children (WIC), 302

Y
Yogurt
 Greek, 92
 Parfait, 106

Z
Zinc, 250

Made in the USA
Middletown, DE
10 March 2025